yinYoga Principles & Practice

yin Yoga Principles & Practice

10th ANNIVERSARY EDITION

paul grilley

White Cloud Press
Ashland, Oregon

Inquiries should be addressed to:
White Cloud Press
PO Box 3400, Ashland, Oregon 97520.
Website: www.whitecloudpress.com

Book Design: Confluence Book Services
Photography: Bruce Bayard
Illustrations: Ann DiSalvo

First edition: 2002
  17 18 19 20   13 12 11 10 9

Printed in the United States

Library of Congress Cataloging-in-Publication Data

Grilley, Paul, 1958-
 Yin yoga : principles and practice / Paul Grilley. --
10th anniversary ed.
    p. cm.
 Includes bibliographical references.
 ISBN 978-1-935952-70-1 (pbk.)
 1. Yin yoga. I. Title.
 B132.Y6G678 2012
 613.7'046--dc23
                                        2012027786

Contents

Foreword   ix

Prologue   xi

1   Ancient Science of Yoga   1

2   Yin and Yang Yoga   12

3   How to Practice Yin Yoga   19

4   Designing Your Practice   30

5   An Outline of Yin Yoga Postures   37

6   Sitting   90

7   Chakra Theory   100

8   Bandha Practices to Awaken Shakti   111

9   Pranayama Practices   122

10   Meditation   126

Bibliography   131

Appendix   139

About the Author   141

This book is dedicated to my teachers,

Dr. Garry Parker, who taught me anatomy,
Paulie Zink, who taught me Taoist Yoga,
Dr. Hiroshi Motoyama, whose work demonstrates
the unity of Taoist and Tantric practice.

Acknowledgements

I would like to thank my beautiful wife Suzee for posing and for the countless hours of discussion, Ann DiSalvo and Bruce Bayard for their artwork, Steve Sendar and Christy Collins of White Cloud Press for their support, and most especially Steve Scholl of White Cloud Press, who insisted this book be created in spite of my hesitations, I owe him a great debt.

Foreword

It has been ten years of study, teaching, and practice since the first edition of this book, much of which is reflected in this second edition. I have expanded the psychological and theoretical descriptions of yin yoga and have tried to better prepare the student about what to expect when practicing. The meditation section has been completely rewritten and the practices elaborated in systematic detail. I have tried to show that controlling one's chi is the thread that leads from physical to emotional and spiritual development.

Whatever form of yoga the reader prefers, I hope she finds the outline of principles presented here useful to her future studies.

Prologue

It was never my intention to promote yin yoga as an independent system of asana practice because yin yoga is, by definition, incomplete. It was and is my intention to promote yin yoga as a supplement to yang forms of exercise. Yang exercise is a broad term meant to include not just yang forms of yoga but any form of exercise that focuses on moving the blood and exercising the muscles; examples include weightlifting, running, cycling, and swimming.

Yin and yang forms of yoga balance each other. The meridians in our body can be favorably compared to irrigation canals: yin forms of yoga dredge the canal of accumulated debris, and yang forms of yoga stimulate the flow of fluid through them.

Yin and yang forms of yoga also balance us emotionally and mentally. Yin yoga soothes and calms us, yang yoga invigorates and refreshes us. Each form of exercise is needed at different times. The modern world is very yang; life should be a balance between competition and compassion, between ambition and contentment, but this balance has been lost. An overemphasis on yang qualities has polluted the planet, split our families, and emptied our homes while both parents work to get ahead or just to stay afloat. Yin yoga can help bring balance to an overly yang lifestyle.

It hasn't always been the case that yang is overemphasized. In some communities the opposite has been the case. In past times "monk's disease" was a colloquial expression used to desribe someone who was overly sensitive to any disturbance. The antidote to monk's disease is yang activity, which is reflected in the fact that hatha yoga, kung fu, chi gong, tai chi, and other yang forms of exercise originated in monastic communities. I have recently heard of a psychotherapist specializing in depression who won't accept clients unless they commit to a regular exercise program. Yin and yang are necessary aspects of a healthy life.

Any skill requires deliberate practice. This is as true of cultivating an inner calm as it is of becoming outwardly athletic. Yin yoga can help. Learning to stay in a pose for five minutes at a time trains the mind and body to become calm and endure distraction, both physical and mental. I took up the practice of yin yoga to cultivate greater flexibility in my joints, but what I discovered is a style of yoga that cultivates physical ease and mental calm. I have long abandoned my ambitions for greater range of motion, but the deeper qualities of yin yoga have kept me practicing for over twenty years.

Yoga in general is widely popular and socially acceptable. This is a seismic shift from the social norms of fifty years ago. I remember my grandmother telling me, "If you have time to exercise then you have time to work," which was her way of saying my yoga practice was a waste of time. But my grandmother was a product of her generation — she raised a family during the Depression and lived through World War II, the Korean War, the Vietnam War, and the Cold War. Most of her adult life was spent doing the very real work of building up the physical infrastructure of the country she was born in.

My generation, that of the post-World War II baby boom, is heir to the labor and sacrifices of our parents and grandparents. Thanks to their work, we live in a time of material luxury, and many of the physical dangers and diseases that threatened our grandparents seem distant to us. What then will be *our* contribution to the future? I believe part of the answer is to live noble lives, lives of kindness and tolerance and gratitude and contentment. But none of these things is possible if we are unable to control our impulses and quiet our minds.

I do not believe that happiness lies in carrying Darwinian survival of the fittest to its extreme. I do not believe that constant accumulation is the proper goal of a human being. I do believe, however, that it is noble and proper to voluntarily trace a circumference around our desires and to deliberately increase the time we spend cultivating kindness, tolerance, gratitude, and contentment. If my generation can pass down practical techniques that cultivate these qualities, then I think we have fulfilled part of our responsibilities to the next generation.

Three Threads of Recent History

What is yin yoga, and how did it get its name? This book is dedicated to three people who represent the three threads that are woven into yin yoga. The first is Dr. Garry Parker. Dr. Parker taught me anatomy and encouraged my first attempts at teaching yoga at Flathead Valley Community College in 1980. From him I learned to appreciate the scientific principles of human movement. It was because of him that I acquired the concepts and vocabulary to competently study anatomy on my own. My view of yoga was shaped by anatomy from the beginning, and I will always be grateful for this.

The second person in this story is Paulie Zink. Paulie is a martial arts expert and teacher of Taoist Yoga. Paulie taught me the basics of Taoist Yoga in 1989.

I first saw Paulie being interviewed on a public access talk show dedicated to the martial arts. At first I was impressed by his gentle and restrained answers to the questions put to him. He seemed to have none of the arrogant swagger or challenging stare of other martial artists I had met. Then he gave a brief demonstration of the yoga that was the foundation of his martial arts training. I was very impressed.

I contacted Paulie and he graciously invited me to join his weekly class on Taoist Yoga. Paulie practiced poses for five to ten minutes at a time, chatting contentedly as he led the class. After nearly two hours of floor poses we would stand and do some moving yang forms that imitated the movements of animals. It was all very interesting and all very different from the hatha yoga I was teaching.

I stopped training with Paulie after about a year. By then I understood the simple principles of yin yoga. I had practiced some of his yang forms and had even dabbled in some of his kicking and punching exercises, but my interests were the floor poses, and it seemed inappropriate to take up Paulie's time when he had several students who wished to learn all aspects of the Taoist Yoga he had to offer.

When I started to teach long floor postures in my public classes the studio owners wanted to know what to name the style in their advertising. Even though I included many traditional hatha yoga postures in my classes, the long, slow holds were certainly different from what everyone else in the studio was teaching, so out of respect for Paulie Zink I suggested "Taoist Yoga." And that was the name I used for ten years.

The third person in this story is Dr. Hiroshi Motoyama. Dr. Motoyama is a Shinto priest and has doctorates in philosophy and physiological psychology. He has demonstrated objectively the existence of both chakras and meridians in experiments. I was drawn to Dr. Motoyama after reading an early work of his entitled "Theories of the Chakras." My wife and I have been students of Dr. Motoyama since 1990. We have visited with him many times both in Japan and at his graduate school in Encinitas, California. Our own yoga and meditation practices have been profoundly influenced by his work.

Dr. Motoyama has demonstrated that the meridians of acupuncture are water-rich channels in the connective tissues that interpenetrate all the structures of the body. Of this theory we will have more to say later, but for now it is enough to say that it confirms ancient theories and illuminates why the system of yoga postures was developed and how they work.

Sarah Powers and How Yin Yoga Got Its Name

The three threads of yin yoga are the anatomy I learned from Dr. Parker, the practice I learned from Paulie Zink, and the meridian theory of Dr. Motoyama. But none of this would be of interest to very many people if not for Sarah Powers.

In the year 2000 my wife Suzee and I presented a workshop on Taoist Yoga in Berkeley, California. Sarah and Ty Powers were part of that small group. We had become acquainted years before in Los Angeles, but Suzee and I had moved to Ashland,

Oregon in 1994 and Sarah and Ty had relocated to the San Francisco area. Sarah attended our workshop because she was interested in revisiting the Taoist Yoga she had experienced in my classes in the early 1990s.

After that Berkeley workshop Sarah resumed her busy traveling and teaching schedule. She began introducing long, slow poses into her classes, explaining that the flowing standing poses were the yang of her practice, and the long floor poses were the yin. When students asked where they could get more information about the yin practice, Sarah graciously referred them to me. I started to get inquiries from studio owners asking me to come and present "yin yoga" workshops, and I gladly accepted. A year later I thought it would be convenient to have my spiral-bound manual on "Taoist Yoga" professionally printed by White Cloud Press. It seemed inappropriate to publish it as "Taoist Yoga" since a book with that name should outline both yin and yang training, so we published the book as *Yin Yoga: Outline of a Quiet Practice*.

Is Yin Yoga New?

Yin yoga is not new. It is a descriptive term that was coined to differentiate between this softer, more traditional style of yoga and the modern vinyasa styles of yoga. To understand the need for making this distinction, we need a brief history of yoga's last thirty years.

Hatha yoga has been a part of American physical culture since the 1890s, but it had never been very popular. Mainstream America either thought it was bizarre or suspected it was a subversive practice taught by Hindu evangelists. Exercise instructors were bored by it because it had none of the movements or muscular effort demanded by the calisthenics they were used to teaching. This is because, with few exceptions, hatha yoga was taught as a gentle system of static, standing poses followed by gentle floor poses followed by gentle breathing exercises. In other words, yoga was yin. Yoga had found acceptance by the 1970s, but even as late as the 1980s yoga was still a distant last place in popularity when compared to aerobics, weightlifting, and any form of sport. But this was about to change in a big way. A very yang, very strong, sexy, sweaty, muscular wave of yoga was about to crash onto the West Coast of the U.S. and sweep all things before it.

The rise in the popularity of yoga today has been driven by the many hybrids of the Ashtanga Vinyasa system taught by Pattabhi Jois. The gentle yoga of earlier decades was submerged in an ever multiplying number of flowing "vinyasa" styles. There were and still are a variety of yoga styles ranging from the yin of restorative yoga to the yang of ashtanga vinyasa, but it is the hot and muscular styles of yoga that have attracted so much attention from mainstream exercise culture.

I learned ashtanga in 1985 from David Williams. David had first learned the gentle yoga of the 1960s and then went to India to learn more. While in India he witnessed a public demonstration of gymnastics that was so interesting he asked what tradition it was from. He was told, "It is a style of yoga." David looked at the acrobatic movements and nonstop flow of poses and said aloud "That's not yoga!" David's reaction sums up how big a change was about to occur in the yoga world.

Starting in the late 1970s and early 80s, yang yoga styles inspired by ashtanga vinyasa became so popular so quickly that when I started teaching yin classes in 1992 people thought it was something new. The popularity of yang yoga classes continues, but there is a growing interest in yin forms of yoga as well. This is inevitable—yin and yang must eventually balance each other in every aspect of life, including exercise.

Most yogis, even the most dedicated yang yogis, eventually develop a yin practice on their own. I have rarely presented a workshop on yin yoga where someone did not say "I have practiced yoga like this for years but didn't give it a name." Yin yoga is a natural, healing practice that talented yoga teachers have always been rediscovering and integrating into their practice.

CHAPTER 1 Ancient Science of Yoga

Three Bodies

From ancient times yogis have postulated that there are three levels of human embodiment:

1. A causal body of thought and belief.
2. An astral body of emotion and desire.
3. A physical body of material substance.

Spiritual adepts assert that our consciousness is not limited to these embodiments and that with systematic practice we can free ourselves from them and experience a union with all things in the universe, a union that is fulfilling beyond anything our presently limited existence can offer.

Three Pillars of Yoga Theory

The systematic practices that slowly disentangle our consciousness from our three bodies are collectively referred to as the science of yoga. All sciences have a theoretical and a practical aspect. These are the three main pillars of the theory of yoga:

1. Our three bodies are knit together and influence each other through special centers in the spine and brain called Chakras.
2. The energy that flows through these chakras is called Chi.
3. This energy flows through our bodies in channels called Meridians.

The fundamental goal of taoist and tantric yoga is to unite our awareness and chi and guide them into our chakras. As we become more skilled in this endeavor we become more conscious of our emotional attachments and mental misconceptions. If we can patiently dissolve these knots, then our energy and consciousness can slip free of all three bodies and expand into realms of unimagined wisdom and bliss.

Three Dimensions of Chi

A yogin who sits to meditate will become absorbed by one of three manifestations of chi: physical, astral, or causal.

The manifestation of chi in the physical dimension is awareness of some part of the body or a pleasant sensation of energy flowing through the meridians. If this flow is blocked then the yogin experiences discomfort.

The manifestations of chi in the astral dimension are memories and desires. The content of these memories or the nature of these emotions can be surprising and shocking. This is because they are manifestations of our unconscious mind that we usually suppress and try to reject. Other memories and desires are less shocking, but all bring with them strong emotional content that needs to be examined if we are to be free of them.

The manifestations of chi in the causal dimension are much subtler than either the physical or astral dimensions. As meditation deepens, the yogi becomes aware of the fundamental ideas that form her or his personality, such as religious beliefs or ideas of social justice. Becoming aware of these beliefs will not destroy them, but it allows the practitioner to understand why she or he has them, which provides the power to dissolve, modify, or retain them.

Two Traditions, One System

According to several ancient views of cyclic time the world entered a period of spiritual darkness around 800 BC. Prior to this descent, the civilizations of India and China had produced wonderful works of art and science, but this dark age brought about their destruction as humans became brutish, selfish, and shortsighted. Ignorance and intolerance led to more and more schools being closed, temples being sacked, and libraries being burned. What fragments of learning survived to the present age are the shipwrecked remains of once well developed sciences. Nonetheless, the skeletons of these ancient theories are basically sound and modern science is on the verge of reanimating them.

Two systems of medical energetics have come down to us from those dark ages: the Indian Tantric and the Chinese Taoist traditions. In Tantra the energy is called prana. The centers that control prana are called chakras, and the channels in which prana flows are called nadis. In Taoism the energy is called chi. The centers that control chi are called dantians, and the channels in which chi flows are called meridians.

The descriptions of nadi-channels in tantric texts are very sparse, but the descriptions of the chakra-centers are very detailed. It is the opposite with taoist texts: the descriptions of meridian-channels are very detailed, but the descriptions of the dantian-centers are sparse. So we use the tantric term when referring to the chakras, but we use the taoist terms chi and meridians. This is a deliberate attempt to present these two traditions as different descriptions of the same system.

Dr. Hiroshi Motoyama has painstakingly detailed the correspondences between taoist and tantric descriptions of chakras, chi, and meridians, and I recommend his book Theories of the Chakras to the interested reader.

Old Wine, New Bottles

The taoist yogis of China based the science of acupuncture on their subtle spiritual perception of chi moving through meridians. They developed breathing and meditation techniques to move this chi into their spines and slowly dissolve the knots tying their consciousness to their three bodies. But sitting and meditating for long hours is very hard on the body and causes the chi to stagnate and create painful distractions, so taoist yogis developed exercises to harmonize the flow of chi and heal the body, making it easier to meditate longer. These exercises were later codified into systems like Tai Chi Chuan and Kung Fu. Indian yogis also developed postures and exercises to prepare the body for the rigors of meditation and to gain control over the chi flowing through the meridians. These techniques were later codified into systems of hatha yoga. Our modern cities are now honeycombed with yoga studios filled with people practicing and enjoying the benefits of these ancient systems, but they might be surprised to learn that the theoretical foundations on which they were built have been dismissed by modern science. That is, perhaps, until now.

Modern Meridian Theory

Dr. Motoyama is a Shinto priest and a double PhD scientist who has from an early age practiced the religious austerities of the ancient Shinto religion as well as the meditation practices of Indian yoga. Basing his research on his own intuitive perceptions as well as his scientific studies of other spiritual practitioners, Dr. Motoyama has for the last forty years been documenting the existence of a system of energy channels in the body. Using modern electronic instruments Dr. Motoyama has demonstrated that this energy flows through water-rich channels in the connective tissue. What is more, the behavior and location of these channels are in close agreement with the ancient descriptions of meridians.

If the insights of Dr. Motoyama are correct, then what textbooks have been calling connective tissue is in fact a living matrix that conducts life-giving energy to every tissue, cell, and organ in the body. I refer to this theory as the Modern Meridian Theory.

Connective Tissue

Connective tissue is not what we thought it was. That is the message of the last three Fascia Research Congresses held in Boston, Amsterdam, and Vancouver in 2007, 2009, and 2012. Scientists at these congresses have presented a large number of studies that detail how connective tissue is an electrically conducting, water structuring, contracting and expanding structure that regulates how cells function. All of this research is directly and indirectly corroborating, correcting, and expanding Dr. Motoyama's Modern Meridian Theory.

Every organ, muscle, and bone in our bodies is formed by a framework of sponge-like material called connective tissue. All of our 100 trillion cells are nested within the spaces of this elaborately interconnected system of pockets and tubes.

Dr. James L. Oschman summarizes the current view of connective tissue and meridians as follows:

> The connective tissue and fascia form a mechanical continuum, extending throughout the animal body, even into the innermost parts of each cell. All the great systems of the body—the circulatory, the nervous system, the musculo-skeletal system, the digestive tract, the various organs—are ensheathed in connective tissue. This matrix determines the overall shape of the organism as well as the detailed architecture of its parts. All movements, of the body as a whole, or of its smallest parts, are created by tensions carried through the connective tissue fabric. Each tension, each compression, each movement causes the crystalline lattices of the connective tissues to generate bioelectric signals that are precisely characteristic of those tensions, compressions, and movements. The fabric is a semiconducting communication network that can convey the bioelectric signals between every part of the body and every other part. This communication network within the fascia is none other than the meridian system of traditional Oriental medicine, with its countless extensions into every part of the body. As these signals flow through the tissues, their biomagnetic counterparts extend the stories they tell into the space around the body. The mechanical, bioelectric, and biomagnetic signals traveling through the connective tissue network, and through the space around the body, tell the various cells how to form and reform the tissue architecture in response to the tensions, compressions, and movements we make (quoted in *Hara Diagnosis: Reflections on the Sea* by Kiiko Matsumoto and Stephen Birch, p. 164).

What is Chi?

When Dr. Motoyama and other scientists conduct research on the flow of energy in meridians they do not directly measure chi, they measure electrical and chemical changes. So what is chi? Chi is the energy that coordinates the electrical and chemical changes that scientists measure.

An analogy from modern physics might be helpful. When solar energy arrives on Earth and strikes the upper atmosphere, this energy becomes manifest as the movement of air. As these winds of air move over the ocean they create waves of water. When these waves of water crash onto a beach their energy becomes manifest as vibrations in the sand. The energy itself is not made of sunlight or air or water or sand, but it manifests its presence in the movements of these "tissues" of the Earth. In a similar way chi is not electricity or chemistry or emotions or memories or thoughts, but all of these things are manifestations of chi in the different tissues of our three bodies.

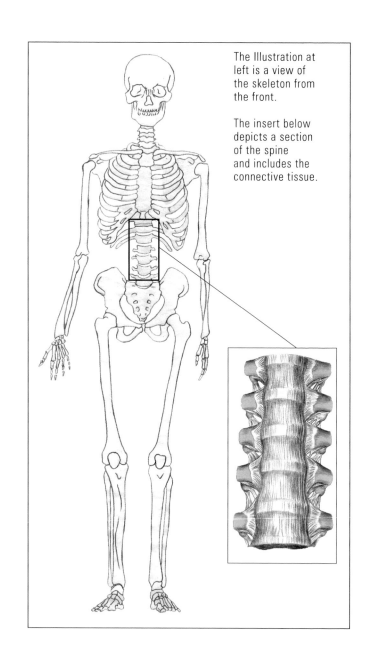

The Illustration at left is a view of the skeleton from the front.

The insert below depicts a section of the spine and includes the connective tissue.

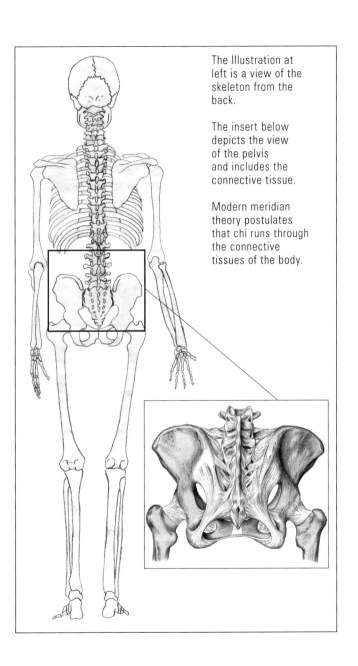

The Illustration at left is a view of the skeleton from the back.

The insert below depicts the view of the pelvis and includes the connective tissue.

Modern meridian theory postulates that chi runs through the connective tissues of the body.

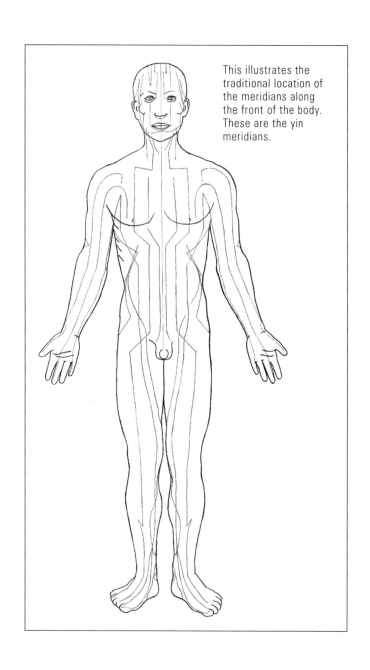

This illustrates the traditional location of the meridians along the front of the body. These are the yin meridians.

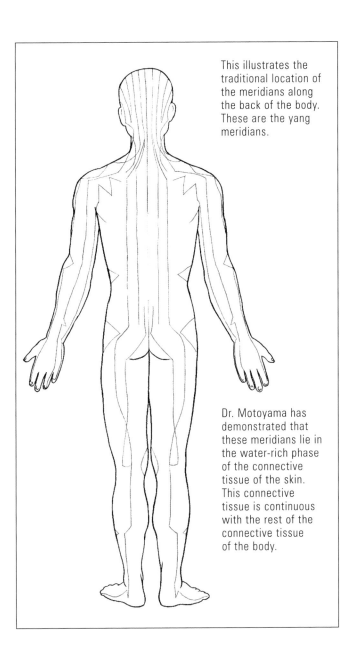

This illustrates the traditional location of the meridians along the back of the body. These are the yang meridians.

Dr. Motoyama has demonstrated that these meridians lie in the water-rich phase of the connective tissue of the skin. This connective tissue is continuous with the rest of the connective tissue of the body.

CHAPTER 2 Yin and Yang Yoga

Yin and Yang

To incorporate modern meridian theory and its insights into our yoga practice we must reacquaint ourselves with the taoist concepts of yin and yang. Yin and yang are descriptive terms that are used to describe all levels of phenomena. Yin is the stable, unmoving, hidden aspect of an object. Yang is the changing, moving, revealing aspect of an object. These two aspects always coexist — there is never one without the other. Everything can be described in terms of its yin and yang; stones, horses, the body, life, thoughts — all have yin-yang aspects.

The following table of examples may help clarify the conception of yin-yang polarities:

YIN	YANG
hidden	exposed
dark	light
cold	hot
still	moving
downward	upward
Earth	Heaven
calm	excited

Yin and Yang are Relative

Yin and yang descriptions of any object are relative. The description varies as different aspects are considered. For example, when considering location, the heart is yin to the breastbone because it is more inside, more hidden. But when considering movement, the heart is yang to the breast bone because it is more mobile.

It can be difficult to determine which aspect of an object should be called yin and which should be called yang. For example, a room is made of walls and the space the walls enclose. We could say the walls are yin because they are solid and the space is yang because it is empty, or we could say the walls are yang because they are what we see and the space is yin because it is not directly perceivable. Even though it is troublesome to determine which is yin and which is yang it is not difficult to appreciate that walls and space are "yin-yang" to each other.

There is no single style of yoga that can be called "yin." All styles of yoga can be described in yin-yang relation to each other and this categorization will change depending on which aspect of yoga practice is considered. If we are basing our distinction on movement-stillness, then the style with the most movement is yang. But if we are basing our distinction on effort-ease, then a strong series of static inversions might be more yang than a gentle, flowing style of yoga. Context is everything and in this book our context is the elasticity of tissue.

Muscle Tissue is Yang, Connective Tissue is Yin

All forms of yoga can be described as yin or yang based on which tissues of the body they target. A practice that focuses on exercising muscles and moving blood is yang. A practice that focuses on connective tissue is yin.

When we move and bend our joints doing yoga postures, both muscle and connective tissue are being stretched. The muscles are yang because they are soft and elastic, while the connective tissues are yin because they are stiff and inelastic. To illustrate the different elasticity of these two tissues, imagine carving a turkey. The actual "meat" of the drumstick is muscle; the "gristle" at the joint which must be cut through or snapped off is connective tissue.

Based on the earlier presentation of the all-pervasiveness of connective tissue, it might seem confusing to distinguish between "connective tissue" and "muscle." It is true that there is no such thing as "just muscle," but the connective tissues that make up muscle are intermixed with other fluids and proteins that give muscle its characteristic elasticity. In a similar way the tendons that bind muscle to bone and the ligaments that bind bones to each other have different elastic characteristics. For our purpose the word "muscle" refers to muscles and their tendons, and the phrase "connective tissue" refers to ligaments and fascia (broad bands of connective tissue).

Yang Yoga Focuses on Muscle

The fundamental characteristic of yang exercise is rhythmic movement. All forms of yang exercise, such as running, weightlifting, and swimming, alternately contract and relax the muscles. Muscle tissues respond very well to rhythmic yang exercise. Most popular forms of yoga—ashtanga vinyasa or power yoga—are yang. They emphasize rhythmic movement and muscular contraction. Most dancers, martial artists, and gymnasts also develop their flexibility with repetitive, rhythmic, yang stretches.

Muscles are bundles of tubes filled with fluids, mostly water. Muscles are up to 90 percent water during intense exercise. The elasticity of muscle tissue varies dramatically with its fluid content—much like a sponge. If a sponge is dry it may not stretch at all without tearing, but if a sponge is wet it can twist and stretch a great deal. Most yoga students like to warm up by doing a series of muscular standing postures or inversions because working the muscles fills them with blood and makes them more elastic.

Exercising muscles also helps bones stay healthy because when muscles vigorously pull on bones the bones respond by becoming thicker and stronger. This is how a forensic anthropologist can determine if she is examining the skeleton of a sedentary aristocrat or a peasant who labored all his life. This is also why vigorous, not gentle, exercise is prescribed to prevent osteoporosis.

Yin Yoga Focuses on Connective Tissue

Exercises that create a gentle traction of the connective tissue are yin. As important as it is for our physical and mental well-being to be strong, it is not muscular strength that gives us the feeling of ease and lightness in the body, it is the flexibility of the joints. I have known many muscularly powerful adults who are physically incapacitated or uncomfortable because of joint problems in their back or legs. Athletes don't retire because of muscular problems, they retire because of joint problems. Bad ankles, bad backs, bad knees—these are the injuries that force athletes to retire and old people to shuffle around. Yin yoga postures gently stretch and rehabilitate the connective tissues that form our joints.

Yin forms of exercise seem new to our way of thinking. People accept the fact that muscle tissue shrinks or grows in response to exercise but imagine that the connective tissues of the body are inert and unchanging. This is not true. All the tissues of the body are changing and adapting to the stresses put upon them.

If we never bend our knees or stretch our spines, the connective tissue is going to shorten to the minimum length needed to accommodate our movements. If we try, after years of abuse or neglect, to flex our knees or bend our spines, we won't be able to do it because our joints will have been shrink-wrapped by the shortened connective tissue. If we want to maintain our joints flexibility, we must exercise them. But we should not exercise them like muscles, we must exercise them in a yin way.

Isn't Stretching the Joints Bad?

Moderately stretching the joints does not injure them any more than lifting a barbell injures the muscles. Both forms of exercise can be done recklessly, but neither is innately wrong or dangerous. Of course, if someone bounces into their joints they will hurt themselves sooner or later, but bouncing is a yang activity, and yin connective tissue shouldn't be trained that way.

Our teeth, for example, are anchored in bone and appear to be immobile. We know from experience, however, that they change. Still, no one would think it viable to "exercise the teeth" by grabbing hold of them and wiggling them back and forth as in yang activity. But with patient, methodical use of braces and retainers, even our teeth can be moved and realigned. Likewise the connective tissues that form our joints can be safely and desirably "exercised" by gently stretching them in yin yoga postures.

Yin and Yang Supplement Each Other

Both yin and yang forms of exercise are necessary, and they supplement each other. Consider as an example the modern medical practices of traction and weight training in physical rehabilitation. People with broken limbs and injured necks are frequently put in traction to relieve stress on fragile bones that are trying to knit together. Once the bones have healed, physical therapy might include weight lifting to strengthen the muscles. This is an example of how yin and yang principles are intelligently employed to recover joint mobility. Traction is the yin principle of static, elongating stress applied for a long time. Moving the neck against resistance is the rhythmic yang aspect of strengthening the muscles.

View of the spine and
pelvis from
the front.

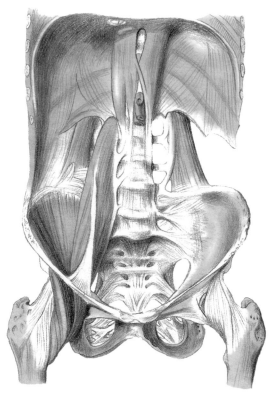

This picture illustrates how the yin and yang tissues
overlay the bones of the skeleton. The white areas
are the deep, yin connective tissues that bind bone
to bone. The dark areas are the superficial, yang
muscle tissues that contract and move.

CHAPTER 3 How to Practice Yin Yoga

The Theory of Exercise

All tissues of the body must undergo stress to stay healthy. If we do not exercise our heart it will degenerate, if we do not exercise our muscles they will atrophy, if we do not bend our joints they will become stiff and painful. Astronauts living in a weightless environment for a few weeks will lose up to 18 percent of their bone density and 30 percent of their muscular strength. Tissues must be stressed on a regular basis to stay healthy, even if only by gravity. In colloquial English, it is "use it or lose it."

All forms of exercise can be classified as yin or yang based on the tissues they target. Exercises that focus on muscles and blood are yang, exercises that focus on connective tissue are yin. Yang exercise is characterized by rhythm and repetition, yin exercise is characterized by gentle traction.

Short-term and Long-term Effects of Exercise are Opposite

The long-term goal of weight training is to make the muscles stronger, but immediately after a vigorous training session the muscles are weak and exhausted. Weightlifters boast about how much they can exhaust their muscles with expressions such as "My legs were so wasted after squats I could hardly walk to my car." So the short-term effect of weight training is muscle weakness, but after weeks and months of regular training and rest the muscles get stronger.

The long-term goal of aerobic conditioning is lower blood pressure and heart rate but the goal in an aerobics class is to raise one's heart rate and keep it raised for several minutes. Even after class it takes an hour or more for the blood pressure and heart rate to return to normal, but after weeks and months of regular training the resting blood pressure and heart rate drop to lower levels that more than compensate for the higher rates during exercise.

This is the normal training effect: the short-term effects of exercise are the opposite of the long-term effects. The same is true of yin yoga practice. One of the long-term goals of a yin practice are strong, flexible joints. Immediately following a long yin pose, however, our joints can feel fragile and vulnerable. This feeling is brief and should pass after a minute or two.

Yin Postures Should Be Held For a Long Time

Dense connective tissues do not respond to rhythmic stresses the way muscles do. Connective tissues resist brief stresses but slowly change when a moderate stress is maintained for three-to-five minutes. To explain why, we will revisit our analogy of connective tissue as a sponge. To make the analogy more accurate, we must imagine the sponges of our bodies completely soaked with fluids that behave like butter. When the butter is solid the sponge is stiff and hard to bend, but when the butter is melted it is easy to stretch and twist the sponge. This change from stiff butter to melted butter is called a "phase change." Holding a stress on connective tissue for several minutes creates a phase change in its fluids, which results in a lengthening of the tissue and a feeling of ease. This phase change also allows a greater movement of chi through the tissues, which is both pleasurable and promotes healing.

Someone new to yoga will probably experience a phase change during a posture but the physical lengthening might not be very profound. In other words, they will experience a pleasant energetic release even if they do not sink much deeper into the pose. But with persistent practice the fibers of connective tissue will grow and realign to allow for a greater range of motion as well.

Yin Postures Should be Held with Muscles Relaxed

To stress the connective tissue around a joint the muscles must be relaxed. If the muscles are tense then the connective tissue doesn't take the stress. You can demonstrate this for yourself by gently pulling on the middle finger of your left hand. When the left hand is relaxed you can feel the connective tissue of the finger joint stretching at the joint nearest the palm. When the fingers of the left hand are tensed and extended you can feel the muscles resist the pull, but the connective tissue is not being stretched.

The stretching of the knuckle may seem a trivial example but the same principle applies to the knees, hips, and spine: the muscles in these areas must be relaxed if the connective tissue is to be stressed when doing a pose.

Note that it is not possible or even desirable for all the muscles of the body to be relaxed when doing yin poses, but the muscles in the target area must be relaxed. For example, in a forward bend you may want to gently pull with your arms or contract your abdomen to increase the stress along the spine. But the muscles along the spine must be relaxed or the connective tissue will not be stretched.

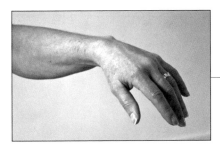 MUSCLES RELAXED

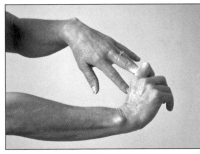 MUSCLES RELAXED

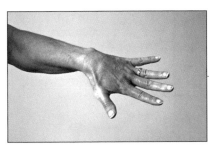 MUSCLES TENSED

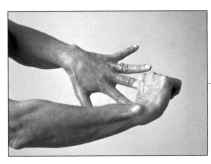 MUSCLES TENSED

HOW TO
PRACTICE
YIN YOGA

Three Layers of a Joint

There are three layers to a joint: the bones, the connective tissue, and the muscles that move the bones. When the muscles are relaxed, the bones can be pulled apart and the connective tissue is stretched. When the muscles are tensed, the bones are pulled tightly together and the connective tissue is not stretched.

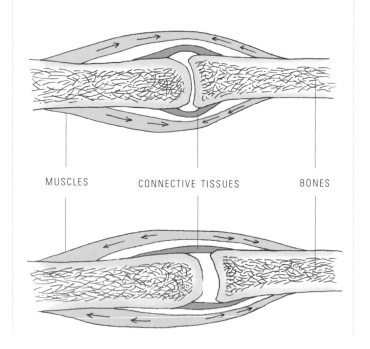

MUSCLES   CONNECTIVE TISSUES   BONES

Yin and Yang Attitude

All things have a yin-yang to them, even our attitude, and one way to illustrate the contrast is by comparing the attitude of a naturalist with that of an engineer. An engineer has a yang attitude, an engineer wants to change things, she wants to tear an old building down or build a new one up, she wants to dam the river or dredge the canal. Her yang attitude is to alter and change what she sees.

A naturalist has a yin attitude. A naturalist wants to know how plants or animals behave without trying to influence them. A naturalist with an interest in butterflies has to go to where the butterflies are and then sit and patiently wait for them to do what butterflies do. A naturalist cannot make butterflies fly or mate or lay eggs, he can only wait and observe. His yin attitude is to try to understand what he is watching.

When practicing yin yoga it is best to have a yin attitude. Do not be anxious or aggressive and force your body into the poses. Make a modest effort to approximate the pose as best you can, and then patiently wait. The power of yin yoga is time, not effort. It takes time for our connective tissues to slowly respond to a gentle stress, it cannot be rushed. Learning to patiently wait calms the mind and develops the necessary attitude for meditation practices.

Modern culture appreciates the strength of the yang attitude to "go for it," but there is no end to our desires. To be truly happy we must also cultivate the yin qualities of patience, gratitude, and contentment.

Yin and Yang Always Coexist

There is no such thing as a pure yin or a pure yang attitude, just as there is no such thing as a pure yin or pure yang yoga practice. These two aspects always coexist. Yin or yang might be dominant in expression but the other is always present.

When practicing a yin pose such as a forward bend, we want to be as relaxed as possible. But if we completely relax every muscle in our body then we might actually fall out of the pose. Some muscular effort is required to balance ourselves in a pose and to maintain the gentle traction, so yang effort is present even in yin yoga poses.

The same can be said of our attitude during yin yoga. It is yin to passively observe the sensations that arise, but it is yang to make the effort needed to maintain the pose.

Breathing

Many beginners unconsciously hold their breath when practicing yoga postures, so teachers often advise them to breathe a certain way to keep them focused yet relaxed. When practicing yin yoga my general advice is to breathe normally. Each posture affects our breathing in a different way. It may be that some postures were specifically designed to alter the breath and thereby alter the perceptions in meditation. To force yourself to breathe the same way in every pose is a yang attitude, and it obliterates the possibility of assessing what the posture does to your natural respiration.

There are times in yin practice when I experiment and hold my breath for a few moments or breathe rhythmically for a little while, but the majority of the time I just passively observe the effect each pose has on my natural respiration.

Feeling the Rebound

After practicing a pose for several minutes it is a good idea to relax on your back and feel the rebound. Poses temporarily block chi and blood from flowing in some areas and redirect it toward other areas. The rebound is what we feel after we release the pose and relax on our backs.

The physical sensations of stretching muscles and joints usually dominates our awareness when we are holding a pose, but when we relax on our backs we can calmly focus on the sensations of chi. This can manifest either as a sense of pressure dispersing away from an area and spreading throughout the body or as a more specific feeling of energy in our spine or legs. After a minute or so the sensations morph and change into a general feeling of peaceful calmness that is not centered in any particular area.

Cultivating awareness of chi is an important part of yoga practice because chi is the thread that ties all three bodies together. Learning to feel chi in the physical body is a first step to objectively experiencing the emotions of the astral body and the thoughts of the causal body.

Rebound and Counter Stretching

The short-term effects of yin practice are the opposite of the long-term. The feeling immediately following a long yin pose is a sense of fragility and vulnerability. Sometimes you can feel a rebounding contraction building up that seems as if it will grow into a painful spasm, but if you stay calm during this process you will find the dreaded painful spasm does not come, and the rebounding wave will reach a crescendo and then subside. This can be a life-changing experience for many people. I have heard from many students who suffered chronic pain for years but healed themselves by learning how to relax in yin yoga.

Some students become alarmed at these sensations and immediately roll to their side or hug their knees or do some other simple counter pose. It is certainly permissible to do counter stretches after a pose, but every once in a while resolve to lie on your back and calmly observe the rebound without reacting.

Exercise in Awareness

Some students say that they "Do not feel anything" when practicing asana or when they are relaxing on their back. This is not possible. There are always sensations arising from our bodies, and we only have to focus our attention to experience them. Our chi will move to wherever we place our awareness. It is also true that wherever our chi moves it will bring our awareness with it.

Try this exercise: Sit comfortably and focus on your nose. Is it warm? Does it itch? Is there a pulse? Is the inhalation in the top of the nostril, or the bottom? Is one nostril more open than the other? Exercises like this are endless and demonstrate the impossibility of being without feeling—we need only direct our awareness to it.

If a student insists he is not feeling something, we can only surmise that he is not feeling what he imagined chi should feel like. It is a misconception to think chi only flows through the meridians depicted on a chart. Chi flows into every cell of the body. The meridians depicted on acupuncture charts are just the surface meridians accessible by needles. There are larger, deeper meridians referred to as "reservoirs of chi." These are the source of the surface meridians. Chi circulates from these deeper meridians into the surface meridians and then back again. The movement of chi in these deeper meridians is felt in the bones, muscles, and organs.

I am not dissuading students from trying to feel specific meridian channels but I am encouraging them not to overlook the more obvious "physical" sensations of chi movement throughout the body and the pleasant calmness it brings.

Learning to Relax

One hundred years ago the American philosopher William James suggested an experiment to illustrate the mind-body connection: Relax on your back and become calm. Once you have succeeded in relaxing, then try to make yourself angry without tensing or altering your body in any way. In other words, try to become angry without tensing your muscles, changing your breathing, clenching your teeth, raising your blood pressure or your heart rate, or manifesting any other physical change. Impossible! Every thought, every emotion puts its imprint on our physical being.

In our highly intellectual, head-oriented world many of us are physically stressed and do not know it. We imagine that by masking our emotions they are not affecting us. But masking suppresses only the crudest outward display of our emotions—our bodies are still taking a beating. If we were more aware of the physical toll of our inner life, we might take more precautions against undesirable mental states.

Learning to relax in poses like the Pentacle helps us to identify and release tensions that are deep within us, not just in the skeletal muscles. Tension in the eyes, jaw, heart, diaphragm, and stomach can be isolated and relaxed. This healthy habit helps us to dissolve the negative tensions that accumulate in our bodies. This is a valuable skill in our heart attack-prone society.

Learning to be Still

Dr. Motoyama has demonstrated that the meridian system and the nervous system are yin-yang to each other. This means that if the energy in one system increases, the energy in the other system decreases. Yin yoga amplifies chi energy and reduces nervous energy; therefore a common reaction after doing yin poses is to desire to just lie still and not move. When deeply relaxed, the effort it takes to move the limbs just doesn't seem worth it.

This inhibition of movement is a desirable state and it is a perfect prelude to meditation. Many people are so nervous they literally cannot sit still for several minutes. A yin practice can change this. If you find yourself wanting to extend your rest phases during your practice, don't fight it. Recognize and enjoy it, and this will develop your ability to recreate the peaceful state of immobilizing inner calm. When you can do this you are nearly over the first hurdle of meditation, which is sitting upright and relaxed for extended periods of time.

CHAPTER 4 Designing Your Practice

Yoga Practice Should Change with Time and Circumstance

Dr. Motoyama once advised me that practicing a specific set of postures for the appropriate period of time could save your life, but that same routine, if continued for too long, could cause great harm. I had this experience with Snail pose. It was my favorite pose for fifteen years, and I did it frequently and for long holds. Then I started having upper spine and ilio-sacral problems which I determined were caused by my favorite pose! I was grieved, but bowed to the truth of experience. I didn't practice Snail for nearly a year, except for some occasional experiments. My symptoms disappeared almost immediately and would return whenever I tried to sneak more Snail into my routine.

After a year I resumed regular five minute Snail poses, but did only one per session and varied my shoulder position each time. I now again enjoy the full spinal stretch and whole body relaxation that Snail brings, but without the spine problems. Why the problems developed I still don't know. The point, however, is that our yoga practice should be alive and adaptable to our needs as we go through the seasons of our lives.

Guiding Principles

As you develop your own sequences of poses, please keep these ideas in mind:

1. Every yoga pose is bad for somebody. Everyone's anatomy and history are unique, and this means that each pose affects each person differently. Usually the difference is trivial, but it can sometimes be significant and harmful. Do not become fixated on "mastering a pose." The poses are meant to be therapeutic, not to challenge your pride. Some poses may be uncomfortable but result in a healthy response, but other poses might just be bad for you.

2. Forward bends are yin. They bring the head level with the heart making it easy to pump blood to the brain. The heart muscle is relaxed and the blood pressure all over the body is reduced. Forward bends harmonize chi flow along the meridians near the spine, which is calming and sedating.

3. Backward bends are yang. They stimulate the nerves and invigorate the yogi. Backward bends do not need to be held as long as forward bends. Experiment with doing more backbends for shorter periods of time rather than longer holds.

4. Time of day and season are important. A more yang practice with shorter holds might be desirable in the morning or on a cold day. A more yin practice might be appropriate in the evenings or on a warm day.

5. The more yang your practice, the greater your variety of poses should be, with shorter durations and more repetitions. The more yin your practice, less variety is needed and the emphasis can be placed on just a few poses.

6. It is fine to practice yang exercise before yin, or yin exercise before yang. Just allow adequate adjustment time when going from one to the other.

7. Use pillows, blankets, and bolsters to support yourself if you find poses stressful. Yin yoga should never be a strain. If you find yourself unable to relax, you are being too aggressive.

Round Spine, Straight Spine

If forward bends are done with a rounded and relaxed spine, then the connective tissues of the torso are stressed more. If forward bends are practiced with a straight spine, then the muscles of the legs are more stressed. Each version of a forward bend has a different emphasis and a yoga student could consider them as two separate poses.

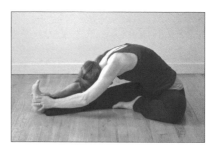

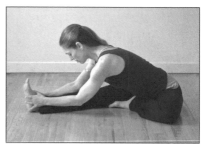

Fixation

Fixation is the vacuum seal that sticks two surfaces together, the most common example being a moist drinking glass set down on a coaster. After a few moments the fluid between coaster and glass is forced out to the sides, and when we pick up the glass the coaster is stuck to it by the vacuum seal. The way to break this fixation is to lift one edge of the glass away from the coaster so that the vacuum seal is broken. This is accompanied with a faint popping sound.

All joints are susceptible to fixation, especially the joints of the ribs and vertebra. These joints have flat, smooth surfaces that are continuously pressed together by gravity and muscle contraction. Sometimes when we bend or twist our spine the bones move enough to break the vacuum seal and create a popping sound. This immediately feels good because the joint can now move more freely and chi flow is increased.

Sacral Fixation

The bone most susceptible to fixation is the sacrum, and once the sacrum fixates it is difficult to move the bone enough to defixate.

In youth the sacrum is inclined forward and helps create the curve of the lower spine, but as we age the sacrum fixates and we unconsciously tuck the pelvis and lose the curve.

Curves reduce compressive stress by flexing front and back. This is why organic things grow in curves—consider, for example, the tendrils of plants or the arches in our feet. This is also why we have curves in our spine. A youthful spine has nice, full curves and easily flexes forward and back. An aged spine has lost its curves and may not flex at all, and this leads to compression of the spinal discs and back pain.

Saddle pose and Caterpillar pose have a yin-yang effect on the sacrum. They are the most effective self-treatment I am aware of for maintaining healthy sacral movement.

Upper-Body Strength

Although this is a book about yin yoga, it is important to say a few words about the yang of upper-body strength. In a taoist analysis of the body, the legs are yin because they are heavier, denser, and closer to the earth. The arms are yang because they are lighter, more mobile, closer to heaven. As we age, the legs become more yin as they become heavy and less mobile. By contrast the arms become more yang, less dense, and less strong. To combat these natural tendencies a yogini should emphasize stretching connective tissue when working the lower body and emphasize muscular strength when working the upper body.

Lower-body posture is influenced most by the flexibility of the sacrum and the curves of the lumbar spine. But upper-body posture is influenced most by muscular strength rather than flexibility.

Failure to do upper-body exercises like Tripod or Crocodile is disastrous for upper-body posture. The muscles become weak, the bones become frail, and the upper spine stoops and rounds.

Three Sample Routines

The following routines are intended to give a beginner a taste of the variety with which the yin poses can be sequenced. There is no one correct way to practice yin yoga. Different people have different needs. I suggest practicing the first routine every other day for a week and make brief notes on how it affects you. Then practice the second routine every other day for a week and make notes. Then repeat this process with the third routine.

Once you are familiar with each routine, I suggest that you practice three times per week, following a different routine each day. Better yet, you might choose to combine a couple poses from each routine and create your own routine of eight to ten poses.

Whatever routine you practice it is important that you relax after each pose. This is the best way to feel what the poses are doing to you. Relaxing between poses is also a good way to not strain anything. Go slowly and enjoy!

First Sample Routine

This first routine is more yang than the others and is focused on the spine's movements rather than the hips. Any or all of the postures can be repeated as many times as needed. If one or two sets is not enough, then do three or four. Just be sure to rest enough and to avoid strain.

1. Leg Raises
2. Snail
3. Caterpillar
4. Tripod
5. Crocodile
6. Camel
7. Child's Pose
8. Saddle
9. Folded Pose
10. Butterfly
11. Spinal Twist
12. Pentacle

Second Sample Routine

This routine focuses on the hips and legs. Any or all of the postures can be repeated as many times as needed. Just be sure to rest enough and to avoid strain.

1. Sleeping Swan or Shoelace on the Wall
2. Half-Frog or Frog on the Wall
3. Dragonfly or Dragonfly on the Wall
4. Swan
5. Half Saddle
6. Folded Pose
7. Caterpillar
8. Spinal Twist
9. Pentacle

Third Sample Routine

This routine is a mix of hip and spine movements. Any or all of the postures can be repeated as many times as needed. Just be sure to rest enough and to avoid strain.

1. Square Pose or Shoelace on the Wall
2. Half Butterfly
3. Caterpillar
4. Dragon
5. Infant
6. Seal
7. Child's Pose
8. Spinal Twist
9. Pentacle

CHAPTER **5** An Outline of
Yin Yoga
Postures

Pentacle

We will start our examination of the yin poses with Pentacle. The reason for this is it is often difficult to feel chi and blood moving in our bodies while we are practicing the poses. The effort required to do them often obscures the subtle sensations. But if we relax in the Pentacle after practicing a difficult posture, then it is quite easy to feel the blood and chi rush into or out of certain areas of our body. Even the discomfort that we feel in the joints we have been stretching is a form of chi and we can learn to observe it objectively. This practice is a great aid to learning to guide the chi when meditating.

Pentacle is done by lying on one's back and spreading the arms and legs out in any comfortable and completely unguarded position. Close your eyes and let the physical body sink into the floor. The ultimate mental yin attitude of mind is to wait without anxiety. Try to feel the various sensations of chi, blood and fluids moving into or out of the parts of the body that were stressed during the previous postures.

The body position as described above is only a suggestion. By spreading the arms and legs, more of the body makes contact with the floor, which is helpful in learning to feel the body, but any relaxing posture will suffice.

Practice Pentacle for one to five minutes or more whenever desired.

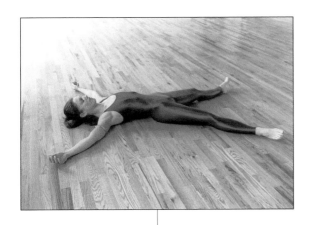

PENTACLE

Half Butterfly

Half Butterfly stretches the back of the straight leg and the spine on the opposite side. It helps to correct imbalances in the flow of chi on each side of the spine. It also helps to decompress the spine, which is valuable in a culture where 80 percent of the population ultimately experience low back problems.

Half Butterfly is done by sitting with one leg stretched forward and the other leg folded with the foot near the opposite groin (A). Drop your chin to your chest, lean forward and try to grasp hold of your ankle or foot (B). Try not to lose your grip as it gives more leverage to the stretch. The knee of the extended leg may be bent a bit in the beginning, but this is fine as long as you feel the stretch along the back of the leg.

Hold this pose three to five minutes.

A

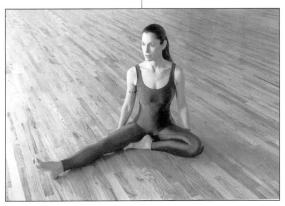

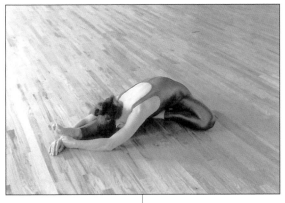

B

Butterfly

Butterfly is a stretch for the lower spine and groin.

Sit with the soles of the feet touching together (A) and lean forward (B). If you start with the feet closer to the groin, the groin muscles are stretched more. If you start with the feet further from the groin, the lower spine is stretched more.

I sometimes suggest this pose to people with very tight hamstrings as it is a good way to stretch the lower spine and doesn't require hamstring flexibility.

Hold Butterfly three to five minutes.

A

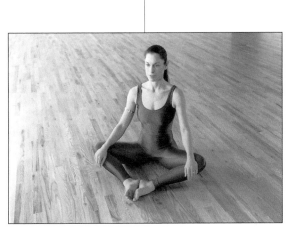

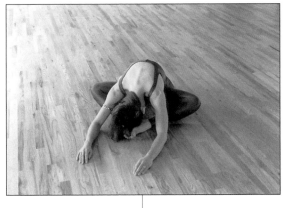

43
AN OUTLINE
OF YIN YOGA
POSTURES

B

Half Frog

Half Frog stretches the hamstrings and the groin. Because the pelvis is pushed forward by the Half Frog position, the stretch on the hamstrings and groin is both easier to achieve and more effective than in Half Butterfly. The beginner will feel the hamstrings more than the groin, but as the student loosens up the groin is also stretched.

Sit with one leg straight and the other leg folded with the foot near your buttocks. The foot of the bent leg may be pointed or flexed (A). Open the legs to a comfortable width and lean forward. If your torso stays over your straight leg, the hamstrings are stretched more (B). If you swing your torso toward the middle of your legs, the groin of the extended leg and the hip of the bent leg are stretched more (C). Be careful not to strain the bent knee.

Hold Half Frog two to three minutes each side.

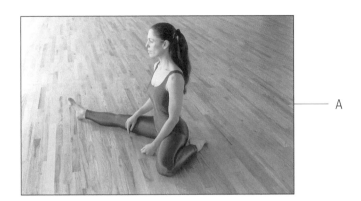

A

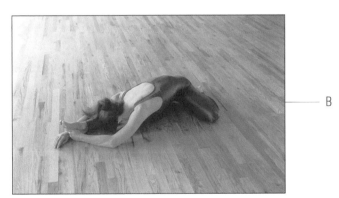

B

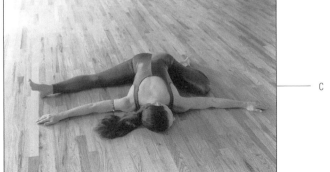

C

Dragonfly

Dragonfly stretches the back of the thighs, lower spine and particularly the groin. This pose can be very frustrating for a beginner as progress seems slow to non-existent. The only advice I can offer is persistence. Stay with it and as you progress in the other forward bends this pose will eventually respond to your efforts as well.

Dragonfly is done by sitting with the legs about 90 degrees or more apart (A) and then leaning forward. Try to touch your hands on the floor in front of you. As your flexibility increases try to rest first your elbows and eventually your head on the floor (B).

Hold Dragonfly three to five minutes.

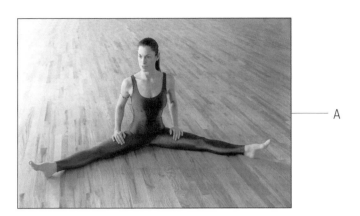

A

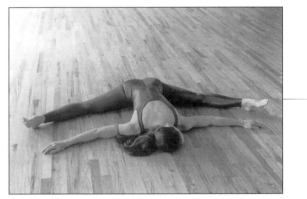

B

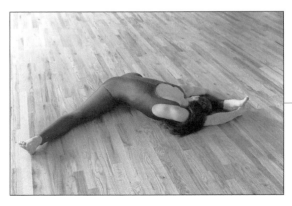

This is a
variation of
Dragonfly.
It gives more
stretch to
the spine and
sometimes the
groin as well.

Sleeping Swan

Sleeping Swan externally rotates the femur of the front leg and stretches all the muscles and connective tissue on the lateral side of the buttock and thigh. It also gently stretches the hip flexors of the rear leg.

Get on your hands and knees and then move your right knee back a foot or so. Move your left foot and place it in front of the right knee (A). Keeping your left foot where it is slide, the right knee backwards as far as possible so your pelvis lowers toward the floor. Lean forward and take some of your weight on your elbows. Your pelvis should be suspended just above the floor with tension in both legs but primarily in the left hip and thigh (B). As you get more flexible you can move the front foot more forward and try to lay on it with your chest.

Hold Sleeping Swan three to five minutes and then change sides.

A

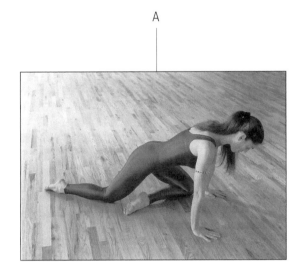

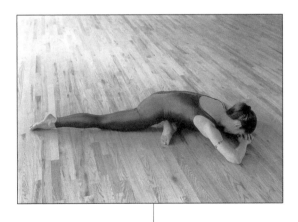

B

Swan

Swan adds a back bend movement to the Sleeping variation. It also stretches the hip flexors of the back leg more effectively. Some students find that it also stretches the front hip better than the Sleeping Swan and so prefer it.

Swan is done by first assuming the Sleeping Swan position and then using your arms to push the torso up and even backward. If you drop your head back, the bend on the spine is increased. When bending backwards, you should experiment with keeping your pelvis down and with letting it twist up as you bend back. These variations will reach into different parts of the spine.

Hold Swan a minute or two each side.

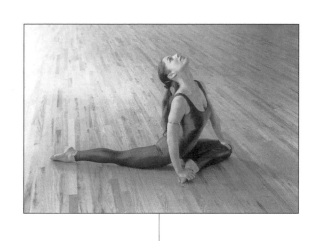

SWAN

Square

Square has much the same effect on the hips and thighs as Sleeping Swan but also stretches the lower spine.

Sit with your legs folded in front of you. Pick up the left leg and try to lay the outer bone of the ankle on top of the right thigh, near the knee (A). Depending on your flexibility, your left knee may be high in the air. You should feel a stretch along the hip and thigh similar to Sleeping Swan. Now try to lean forward. As you do so your chest will push against the left leg and increase the stretch (B). If your hips are loose enough and you can go down further, then you will also begin to feel the stretch along your lower spine.

Hold Square three to five minutes then change sides.

A

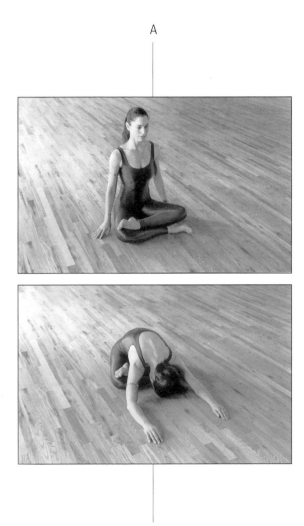

B

Shoelace

A variation of Square is Shoelace. Cross your knees so that they very nearly overlie each other (A) and then lean forward (B). Due to indidvidual differences in anatomy you may prefer Shoelace or Square. Let experience be your guide.

A

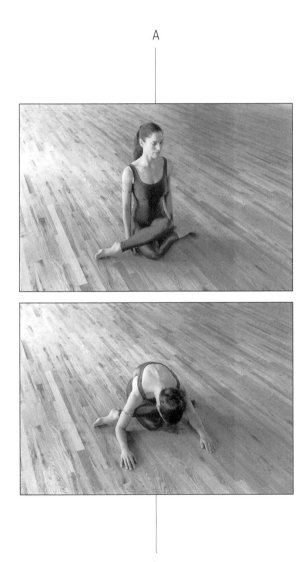

B

Caterpillar

Caterpillar is one of the most basic and important postures. It stretches the legs and the entire spinal column and balances the chi flow. It is a great aid in relaxing the mind and drawing the senses inward, therefore it is a good preparation for meditation.

Caterpillar is done by sitting with both legs stretched out in front of you, feet about hip width apart or narrower if you prefer. Drop your chin to your chest so the muscles and ligaments at the base of the skull are stretched. Now lean forward and try to grasp your ankles or feet. Try to keep your legs straight but don't work too hard. The thighs should be relaxed and a slight bend of the knees is fine as long as you still feel the stretch. Relax the muscles of the legs and spine and feel the stretch move up through the legs and hips and all the way up to the skull.

Try to hold this pose three to five minutes or more.

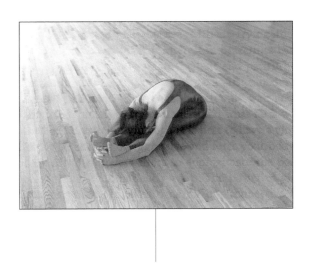

CATERPILLAR

Leg Raises

Leg raises are a muscular (yang) exercise (see page 11). Increasing the flexibility of the lower spine brings with it a greater need for abdominal, lower back (quadratus lumborus) and hip flexor strength. Leg Raises effectively strengthen these areas. Some students, especially after forward bends, also experience wonderful adjustments of their sacrum when performing this exercise.

Lying on your back place your hands under your buttocks, bend your knees and draw them up toward your chest (A). Now try to straighten your legs and lock your knees (B). Lift your chin to your chest and slowly lower your feet toward the floor (C). Stop when your feet are just a few inches off the floor and take a few breaths. This is one repetition.

You should repeat this five times or more.

To vary the training, pause for several breaths with the legs at various heights above the floor. If you tilt your head back, the stress on the lower spine/hip flexor muscles is increased. You can also vary the exercise by bringing the legs up straight rather than bent.

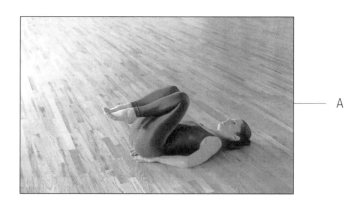

A

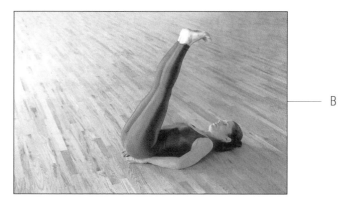

B

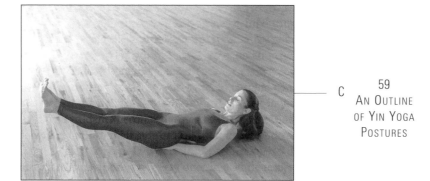

C

Snail

Snail stretches the entire spinal column and induces a withdrawal of energy from external senses and turns the mind inward. Most people, even those for whom this is a difficult pose, find the after effects pleasant.

Snail is done by first lying on one's back with hands under the buttocks and then rolling the legs up over your head (A). Beginners should endeavor to keep the legs straight and may want to use their hands on their hips for balance (B). The feet may not touch the floor but the muscles of the legs and spine will be strengthened and stretched effectively.

After some months the feet should touch the floor at which time you may want to clasp hold of your calves or ankles. Note that at this phase of the Snail you may not want to roll up on your neck but rather keep the hips low and the weight more between your shoulder blades. This version gives a nice stretch to the lower and middle spine as well as the legs (C).

A final variation is to roll up onto the neck and shoulders as much as possible (D), even bending the knees down toward the floor (E). This version is the most strenuous for the neck and upper spine.

Use plenty of padding under your spine and shoulders so the tips of the spinous processes are not bruised. Don't do this pose if you have eaten in the past two or three hours. If it is a struggle for you to roll yourself up into this posture then avoid it for now and continue with Half-forward bend and Forward bend until your spine is more flexible. Women in their period should avoid this pose.

Try to hold Snail one to three minutes or more and then slowly roll down.

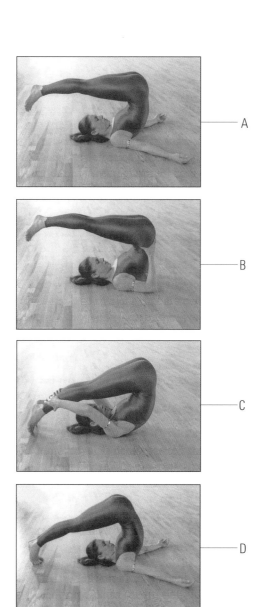

A

B

C

D

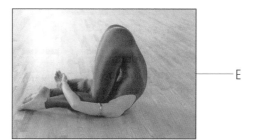

E

Tripod

Tripod is a muscular (yang) exercise, it strengthens the upper body (see pg. 11) and is a wonderful stretch for all the muscles of the torso. It is a nice counter to forward bends and prepares the body for backbends.

Sit up and place your left hand a few feet behind you on the floor. Keep your left leg straight but bend the right knee and place the right foot near your buttocks (A). Using all the muscles of your body, particularly those in your arm and upper back, push your pelvis up as high as possible. Turn to look at the floor while reaching up and over your head with your right hand (B). Stretch your waist and ribs like you're taking a deep yawn.

Hold Tripod one or two breaths and then change sides. Since Tripod is a muscular yang pose I suggest repeating it three times or more.

A

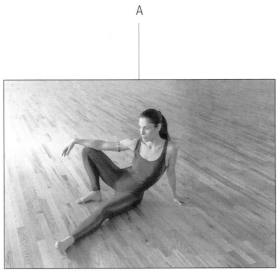

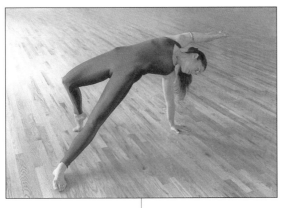

B

Crocodile

Crocodile is a yang, upper body strength posture (see pg. 11). It is the old fashioned push-up. Don't let bad gym-class memories spoil your appreciation of this pose, it is a wonderful way to develope overall body strength and confidence. Although Crocodile is felt most keenly in the arms and shoulders, it develops the strength of the stomach and spine as well.

Starting on your hands and knees, straighten your legs and keep your body perfectly straight (A). Inhale and then exhale and slowly lower your torso toward the floor, keeping your elbows near your ribs (B). Hold this position for a few seconds, inhale and then exhale and push back up to the starting position. As a beginner you may want to do this posture with your knees on the floor until you are stronger.

Repeat three times or more.

A

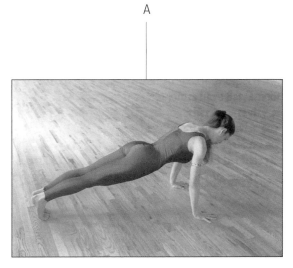

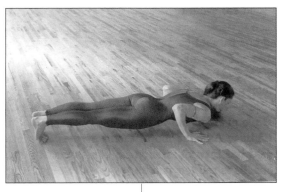

B

Infant

This pose is a yang stimulation for all the muscles along the spinal column. It also stimulates blood circulation in the abdominal organs.

Lie on your stomach with your arms at your side. Now inhale and raise your head and chest up as high as is comfortable. You may or may not want to raise your legs and you may or may not want to keep them together. Follow your instincts as to whatever variations strengthen the spine more.

Hold Infant three to five breaths. Repeat if you like.

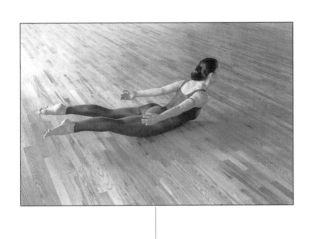

INFANT

Seal

This pose is a strong arch for the lower spine. This is the area of the body where most people are very stiff at best and in pain at worst. Seal works to reestablish a lumbar curve in the spine. This curve is abused and eventually lost by sitting in chairs for hours everyday for years and years. Since most of us will continue to be chair — bound by our jobs, cars, restaurants and social decorum, the need to constantly combat the abuse of the lower spine is ever-present. If you are one of the many who have a "bad back," this posture will be a struggle for quite a while but don't despair, if you gently persist your spine will bend again.

Lie on you stomach as in Infant, with your hands on the floor in front of and to the side of your shoulders. Everyone's body proportions and flexibilities differ so you will want to experiment with exactly where you place your hands. Straighten your arms and raise the torso off of the floor. Turn your hands so the fingers are turned out to the sides, this makes it easier for most people to straighten the arms. The spine and belly are suspended above the floor. Depending on one's proportions and flexibilities, one's pelvis may or may not be lifted above the floor. Some Yogis like to tense the muscles along the spine and others prefer to just "hang" and slowly let the spine form itself into an arch.

Variations of the Seal can effectively isolate different parts of the spine. If you keep your legs apart, the stress in the lower spine will be more pronounced. If you keep your legs together, the stretch is more evenly distributed along the spine. Keeping the buttocks and thighs flexed or relaxed also changes the stress but not in a uniform way for everybody. You will have to experiment for yourself. If you tilt your head back there is more curve placed into the neck and lower spine.

Hold the Seal for a minute and then slowly lower yourself down. Repeat as many times as you feel the need.

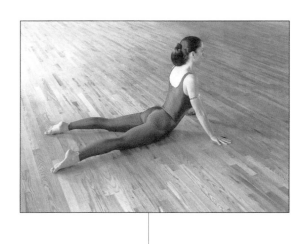

Seal

Child's Pose

This posture gently stretches the spine so it is a natural counter to backbends. It also inclines the head so the heart can rest instead of trying to force blood upward to the brain. If you are feeling cold or vulnerable after practicing postures, then Child's Pose helps.

Child's Pose is done by kneeling with buttocks on heels and folding forward to rest your head on the floor with your arms resting comfortably beside you or in front of you. Close your eyes and empty your mind.

Rest in Child's Pose one minute or more.

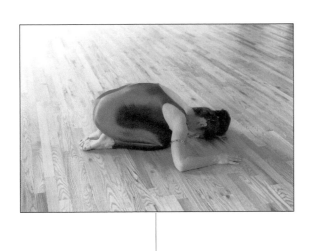

CHILD'S POSE

Dragon

Dragon stretches the groin, ankles, and hip flexors. It also makes backbends easier to do because the pelvis becomes freer in its movements.

Dragon is done by placing one foot forward on the floor in front of you and resting the opposite knee on the floor behind you. Use your hands for balance and slowly lower the thigh of your rear leg to the floor so the top/front of the thigh takes the strain (A). Depending on your flexibility, you might also feel a stretch in the groin of the front leg.

If your stance is not too wide, you can push down on the front knee and exaggerate the stretch on the ankle and achilles tendon (B). If your stance is wide, you will feel the hip flexors on the back leg more (C). Front splits is a variation of Dragon (D).

Try to hold Dragon two or three minutes then change sides.

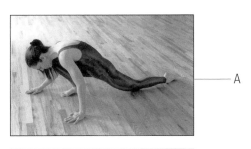 A

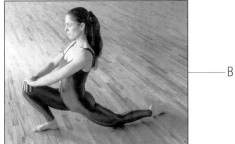 B

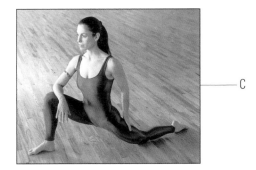 C

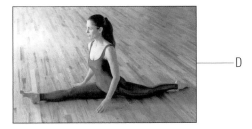 D

Saddle

This pose stretches the feet, knees, thighs, and arches the lumbar and sacral vertebrae.

Saddle is done by sitting on your feet with knees spread apart. For many this is enough stretch for the ankles, knees, and thighs (A). As you become more limber, try to lower yourself backwards and support your weight on your arms. If this becomes easy, go to your elbows. If this becomes easy, arch back and rest the weight on your head (B). If even this becomes easy, you may rest your upper spine on the floor (C). Let the lower spine arch and take the pressure of the bend.

Coming out of Saddle is perhaps more difficult than getting into it. I have consulted many different Yoga books over the years and all advise to just "come up out of the pose." My own experience has been that for many it is less stressful to roll or lean to one side and unfold the legs one at a time. Let experience be your guide.

Try to stay in Saddle one minute and gradually build to three or more.

CAUTION: When people cringe at the thought of over-stressing a joint, this is one of the postures they are thinking of — and for good reason. Foolish aggressiveness or impatience can prove disastrous here. Strong medicine can be strongly abused. It may take years for you to comfortably do the more advanced versions of this pose. Be cautious but don't be para-lyzed with fear. Our chair–bound society with its dangling legs has injured many of us, but basic ranges of motion can be recovered by a sane and patient yoga practice.

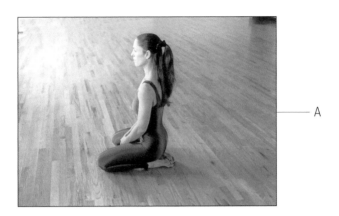

A

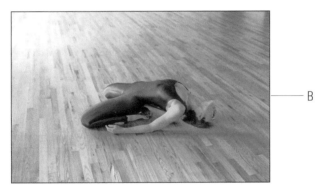

B

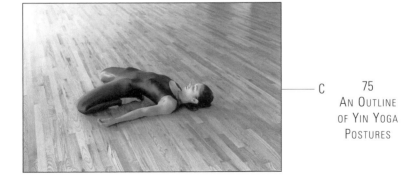

C

Camel

Camel is a variation of, or preparation for, Saddle. If your knees or ankles are too tight to do Saddle, Camel pose will help loosen the thighs and arch the spine. Even if you can practice Saddle effectively, you may like to do Camel as well since the arch in the middle and upper spine is more complete.

Kneeling with knees apart, try to reach back with your hands and support yourself on your feet or calves. Try to keep the pelvis pushed forward and drop your head back.

Try to hold Camel a minute or so.

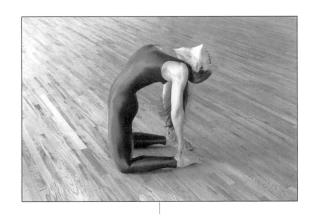

Camel

Half-Saddle

Another variation of Saddle is Half-Saddle. This pose is much like the Saddle but done with only one leg at a time. The arch on the sacro-lumbar spine is less than in the full Saddle but the stretch on the thigh is more.

Half-Saddle is done with the foot resting alongside rather than under the buttock. The free leg can be positioned as one wishes (A or B).

Hold Half-Saddle one to three minutes each side.

A

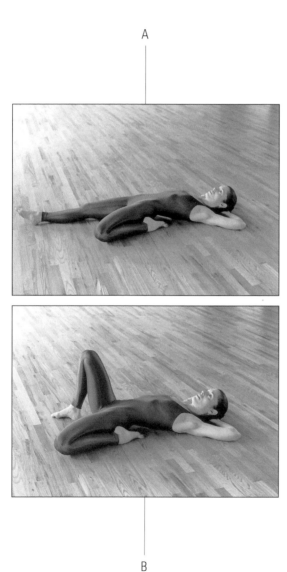

B

Folded Pose

This pose is a gentle stretch for the spine and a mild exercise for the hip joints. It is a nice way to help unwind any tension in the spine from doing backward bends such as Saddle.

Lying on your back draw your right knee to your chest clasping both hands on the knee (A). For a gentle stretch of the upper spine, you may bring your forehead toward your knee as well.

Hold this posture about three breaths, then change sides. After doing each side do both legs together (B).

A

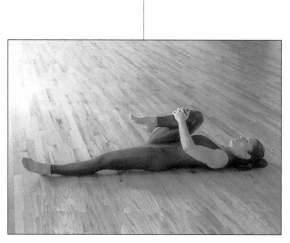

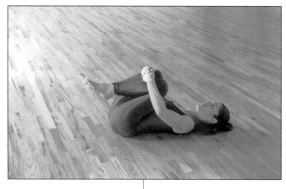

B

Spinal Twist

This pose relaxes tension in the muscles and meridians. It is an excellent pose to end your practice with since it helps relieve any kinks or strains that sometimes occur from Yoga practice.

To do the Spinal Twist, first lie on your back and bring both knees up toward the chest, feet off the floor. Cross the left leg over the right (A), and then twist both legs to the right (B). You may want to lay your right hand over the knees to hold them closer to the floor and you can also turn your head and reach with your left arm to bring the left shoulder closer to the floor and make the twist more complete. How high up you draw your knees varies the twist so you should experiment with different positions.

Hold the pose a minute or so and then change.

A

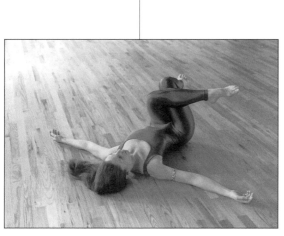

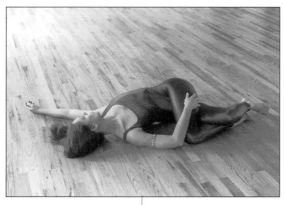

B

Shoelace on the Wall

This version of Shoelace is useful to anyone with tender spines or knees, but even young and healthy yogis like this stretch because it can be relaxing. It is an effective variation of Sleeping Swan, Shoelace, or Square pose.

The target areas of the pose are the muscles and connective tissue on the lateral areas of the buttocks and thighs.

Lie down on your back with your buttocks close to a wall and your legs extended up the wall (A). The closer your pelvis and buttocks are to the wall, the more intense the stretch will be, so adjust your distance accordingly.

Bend your knees to move your feet down and then, bracing yourself with your arms, use your legs to lift your pelvis up off the floor (B).

Place your left ankle just above your right knee, as shown (C). Your right foot is pressed against the wall for the duration of the pose.

Slowly lower your hips (D). This will cause the legs to fold in toward the torso and create a stretch in the buttock or thigh.

Hold Shoelace on the Wall for three to five minutes and then change sides.

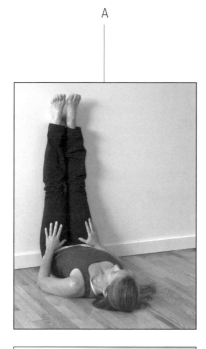

A

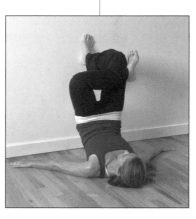

C

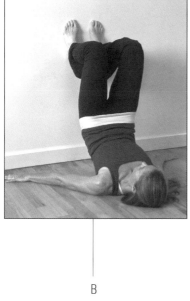

B

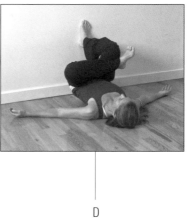

D

Frog on the Wall

This pose is a substitute for either Dragonfly or Half Frog. The target area is the groin muscles.

Lie down on your back with your buttocks close to a wall and your legs extended up the wall (A).

Bend your knees and slide both feet down the wall (B). Then, with a hand on each shin, open your knees and walk your feet out to the sides so that the feet are about the same width as the knees (C). The wider your knees, the stronger the stretch, so adjust your width accordingly. The closer your pelvis and buttocks are to the wall, the more intense the stretch will be, so adjust your distance accordingly..

You might choose to gently rest or press your hands on your knees, but do not force the stretch.

Hold Frog on the Wall for three to five minutes.

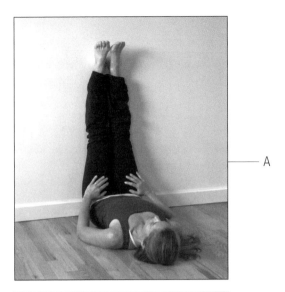 — A

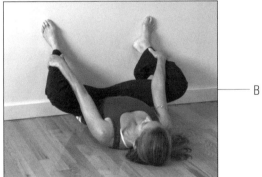 — B

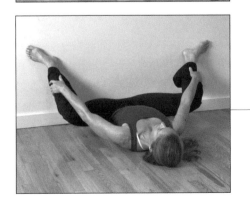 — C

Dragonfly on the Wall

This pose is a substitute for Dragonfly. Its target areas are the groin and hamstrings.

Lie down on your back with your buttocks close to a wall and your legs extended up the wall..

Slowly spread your legs apart and slide your feet down the wall. The wider your legs, the deeper the stretch, so adjust yourself accordingly. The closer your pelvis and buttocks are to the wall, the more intense the stretch will be, so adjust your distance accordingly.

Your legs do not have to be completely straight in the beginning, but as your flexibility increases they will get straighter. Do not rush. It is the stretch that is important, not the aesthetics.

Hold Dragonfly on the Wall for three to five minutes.

A

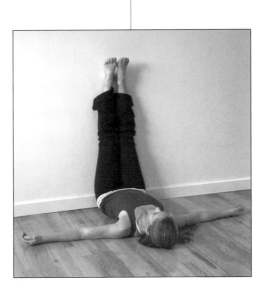

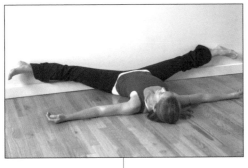

B

CHAPTER **6** # Sitting

Yin Yoga Prepares Us for Sitting

The practice of yin yoga culminates in the ability to comfortably sit in an upright posture for an extended period of time. Until we can do this, our ability to go deep in meditation will be hindered. When most people try to sit they soon become distracted by discomfort in their hips, knees or lower spine. Acupuncture theory says this discomfort is due to the stagnation of chi and blood. The connective tissue in these areas is so tight that the pressure of the posture soon chokes off the flow of chi. A deep yin practice makes these joints more flexible and you will be able to sit much longer before chi stagnation becomes a distraction.

Value of Sitting

The ancient texts on yoga say that proper sitting can heal many diseases. In my own experience this seems possible. My students and I, when sitting for a half-hour or more, have experienced subtle adjustments occurring along the spine. These adjustments or "cracks" along the spine are usually preceded by a slow build-up of pressure at one or two points accompanied by muscle tension over a broader area. When the tension reaches a certain point, a slight twist or adjustment of the body causes the vertebrae and ribs to move with a "cracking" sound and this is accompanied with a wonderful sense of relief or fullness. This whole process might recur once or twice if the Yogi sits long enough. I intuit that these spinal adjustments free the flow of chi to all the body and affect our long — term health.

All of us come to a practice of sitting with some history of injury or neglect of our spines, and learning to sit is going to bring uncomfortable sensations due to spinal misalignments and blocked chi flow. The practice of yin yoga helps minimize these symptoms, but even the most flexible and healthy of us will suffer through some physical discomfort as the body slowly readjusts itself. These symptoms are an inevitable part of spiritual discipline and sometimes recur for even veteran meditators. I mention this to encourage those who labor under the illusion that they are the only ones who find something so "simple" as sitting a difficult thing to do. It is not for nothing that over two thousand years ago Patanjali, the great systematizer of Yoga philosophy, listed learning to sit as one of the essential skills a Yogi must develop.

Tilt of the Pelvis

All sitting postures aim at one thing — a comfortable, upright posture. Straining or slouching in a pose creates uncomfortable pressure points and this interferes with the flow of chi up and down the spine. The most fundamental factor in achieving a comfortable sitting posture is the tilt of the pelvis. The upper body takes care of itself if the pelvis is properly adjusted.

When a person tires while sitting, the top of the pelvis is unconsciously tilted backward. As a result the whole body slouches, the flow of chi is reduced, and in a matter of minutes the would-be meditator gives up. When this person "straightens up," they are tilting the top of the pelvis forward. It is this vertical or slightly forward tilt of the pelvis that establishes a comfortable meditation posture.

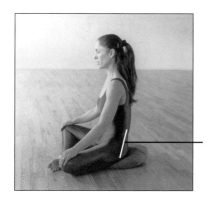

The line in this picture shows a backward tilting pelvis, creating a slouched and uncomfortable posture.

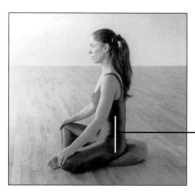

The line in this picture shows a vertical tilt of the pelvis.

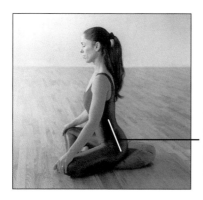

The line in this picture shows a slightly exaggerated forward tilt ofthe pelvis.

Siddhasana

Siddhasana is the most popular of the meditation postures. In Sanskrit it means "the perfected pose." One foot is pulled in with the heel as close as comfortable to the genitals. The other foot is pulled in front of the first. You might want to occasionally alter the foot positions.

The hands should be placed so that the arms and shoulders can rest comfortably. You might rest hands folded together on your lap or on the knees with palms up or palms down. I sometimes assume an asymmetrical position with one hand on my lap and the other palm down on my knee (A).

The key to siddhasana is that the hip joints should be elevated at least as high as the knees, if not higher. If the hips are lower than the knees, then the top of the pelvis will be tilted backwards and this will quickly fatigue the muscles of the lower spine, causing discomfort. Sitting on the edge of a pillow or rolled blanket makes all the difference in being able to sit comfortably as this raises the hips above the knees (B).

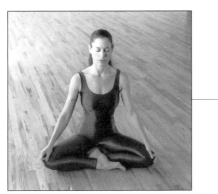

A

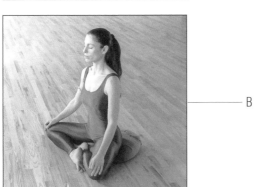

B

Seiza

Seiza is commonly called "sitting Japanese style." It is much like the beginning phases of Saddle except the knees are kept close. The buttocks rest on the heels and the hands rest folded on your lap (A). Very flexible people sometimes sit between their feet rather than on them (B). Either variation is made easier by sitting on a small cushion or folded blanket. This relieves the pressure on the back of the knees and calves. Many bookstores now sell "seiza benches" or "meditation benches" that work much like a cushion (C).

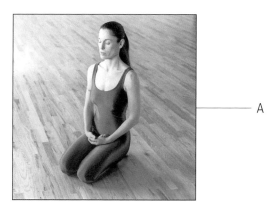 A

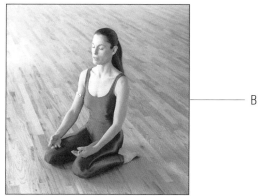 B

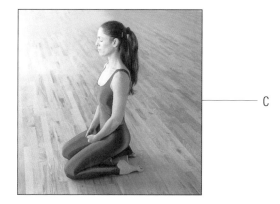 C

Sitting in a Chair

The most accessible posture for Westerners is sitting on the edge of a chair with the spine straight and not touching the back of the chair. This is the posture Paramahansa Yogananda taught to his Western students.

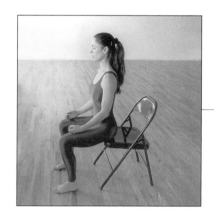

SITTING IN A CHAIR

Chakras within Sushumna

The three pillars of yoga theory are chi, meridians, and chakras. We have explored chi and meridians. We will now elaborate the theory of the chakras.

Chakras are spiritual centers in the brain and spinal cord where the physical, astral, and causal bodies are knit together and influence one another. There are several chakras: some are considered major, some minor. Some traditions focus on five chakras, others focus on nine. In this text we will focus on the seven major chakras.

The chakras are located within a special meridian that lies inside the spine. This meridian is called sushumna. The chakras are strung along sushumna like beads on a string. Sushumna is said to start from the coccyx and reach all the way up to an opening in the top of the skull. The opening in the top of the skull is called the fontanel. It is quite soft in infants and remains that way until the bones of the skull grow together some months after birth. This opening is called Brahman's Gate. Brahman is the name for the Absolute, the source of all creation.

Chakra Location

When trying to describe where a chakra "is," one finds oneself in a dilemma. Common language suggests chakras are physically located in the spine, but the reader should bear in mind that this is both true and false. A "broken heart" is a real experience that indeed seems centered in the heart, but that is not where the feelings actually reside. The chakras have a physical correspondence, but they are more than physical. Bear this in mind when reading about "where" a chakra "is." Don't be limited by only physical conceptions.

Dr. Motoyama writes that chakras might be described as having a root and flower. The roots of a chakra are in sushumna within the spine, but the flower of a chakra opens out from the spine and into the body in a significantly larger but less defined region. Some people are more sensitive to the sensations in the flower region of a chakra, while others are more immediately drawn into sushumna. It is best to focus where you are most sensitive, but don't forget that our experience of a chakra will deepen and change as we progress. Meditating on the root or flower of a chakra is only a starting point.

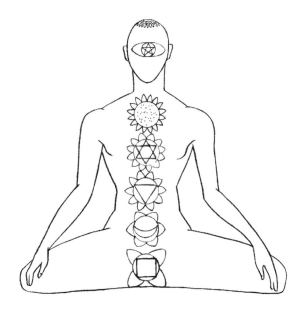

CHAKRA	ROOT	FLOWER
Sahasrara	Top of Brain	Above the Head
Ajna	Center of Brain	Third Eye
Vishuddha	C-7 Vertebra	Throat
Anahata	T-7 Vertebra	Heart
Manipura	L-2 Vertebra	Upper Abdomen
Svadhisthana	Sacrum	Lower Abdomen
Muladhara	Coccyx	Floor of Pelvis

Chakras and the Three Bodies

Our three dimensions of existence constantly interplay with one another. Our causal body of thoughts is of a different dimension than our physical body, but a stirring patriotic speech or outrageous social injustice can impact our physical body very strongly. The same is true of the emotions of our astral body. Our heart rate, blood pressure, adrenalin, indeed all of the systems of the physical body, are altered by our thoughts and emotions. It is also true that altering our physical state affects the astral and causal dimensions.

The causal body gave birth to the astral body which gave birth to the physical body. But we identify so strongly with the physical body that we have become unbalanced in our life's pursuits. All of the vast wisdom of the causal worlds remain unknown to us and the deeper, less selfish emotions of the astral world are not consciously developed. The yogin seeks to expand his or her consciousness into these higher realms by learning to stop the movements of chi as it manifests in each dimension. In the physical dimension, this means sitting still and slowing the breath. In the astral dimension, it means controlling our responses to the emotions we experience. In the causal dimension, it means calmly observing our thoughts without reaction or attachment.

Shakti and Shiva

Fundamental to the theory of the chakras are the concepts of Shakti and Shiva. Shakti is the energy that forms all things and Shiva is the consciousness that guides and coordinates them.

All things in the universe, from atoms and stars to animals and angels, are complex webs of energy coordinated by a guiding consciousness. But the division of things into energy and consciousness is not absolute, only apparent. Shakti must be conscious in some way or it could not respond to the coaxings of Shiva. And Shiva must possess some form of energy or it could not influence Shakti's work. Shakti and Shiva are the ultimate Yin-Yang, the ultimate Female-Male, they do not exist without each other, they are two aspects a single, indescribable Absolute Reality.

Shakti and Shiva in the Physical Dimension

Shakti provided the energy needed to multiply a single fertilized human egg cell into the tens of trillions of cells that comprise our physical body but without Shiva consciousness guiding this process then these tens of trillions of cells would have only been a shapeless, wriggling ball of flesh. It is the power of Shakti that multiplied and grew our cells. It is the consciousness of Shiva that coordinated this growth to form our wonderfully complex and elegant bodies.

As our bodies grew Shakti became less active and She now sleeps in the lowest chakra at the base of the spine. Most of Her power is dormant now, but some of that power manifests itself as the chi circulating through our meridians. After our bodies were formed according to our various karmas, the vast consciousness of Shiva withdrew but left us with an awareness of our physical being and only a dim awareness of our deeper dimensions.

Chakra Purification in the Physical Dimension

The chakras are said to hold the seeds of all our past desires and habits. The function of the chakras is to manifest those desires to our consciousness so that plans can be made and actions can be taken to satisfy them. Yogic theory is that if we had no unfulfilled desires and could uproot our previous habits of behavior, then we could easily slip free of these three bodies. Becoming aware of the karmic seeds stored in the chakras and dissolving them is called chakra purification. We become aware of these seeds by meditating on the chakras. At first our meditation is focused on the physical location of the chakras but as meditation deepens the emotional and causal content of the chakras is revealed to our consciousness.

In the physical dimension, purification is achieved by sitting still and slowly restricting the breath. Chi is consumed by ceaseless, unconscious movement and irregular breathing. Sitting without movement and reducing the breath rate liberates a large amount of physical chi that can then be transmuted by the chakras into energies of the astral and causal bodies. This enables a yogin to consciously explore and develop these dimensions.

Chakra Purification in the Astral Dimension

As her meditations become more profound a yogini will start to experience thoughts, memories, and emotions that are active in the astral dimensions of each chakra. The general term for whatever occupies our conscious field is vritti. Vritti literally means "whirlpool," but in context it means thoughts, memories, and emotions. The yogini meditating on a chakra gradually becomes aware of memories and emotions she did not suspect were there.

At first the vrittis she experiences will be related to her everyday concerns and relationships, but with further practice they become the stronger and more emotionally charged events that have shaped her personality. Re-experiencing these vrittis can be shocking and humbling. They range from early childhood events to being rejected by a lover or being fired from a job. They include naked lusts and shameful moments of lying or cowardice or ingratitude, or being hurt, or being unfairly treated. Although she is rarely conscious of them, these suppressed vrittis will continue to influence her behaviors until they are consciously confronted and dissolved.

Nonattachment

When vrittis arise the yogini should examine them without attachment. She should let them pass through her, not hold on to them or amplify them. But she should not deny them, either. Each time she objectively examines them they will lose some of their emotional energy. When she no longer has a strong reaction to them, they become a new source of strength and wisdom. She will no longer be unconsciously compelled to repeat those behaviors or be plagued by an unreconciled past. She will become truly compassionate and understanding of others, even those who negatively affect her.

Of course not all vrittis are distressing. Some memories and impulses can be a source of strength and comfort, and after a yogini has experienced them she should dismiss them and return to the focus of her meditation.

It is possible the vrittis a yogini experiences are not arising from the chakra she is focused upon. They might be emanating from a chakra that just happens to be more active at the moment. Whichever vritti arises, a yogini should objectively examine it and then dismiss it or follow it to its source.

Chakra Purification
in the Causal Dimension

As our spiritual life deepens, our vrittis will reflect our causal body of beliefs and ideas, beliefs so near to our sense of self that we have never thought to question them. We are more attached to our ideas than our physical bodies. People are willing to die or are willing to kill for their beliefs. In one sense it is noble to die for ideals; in another sense, attachment to our causal ideas can provoke us to commit murder.

Our causal body of beliefs and ideas should not be confused with knowledge of various facts. Even the most ignorant of men have beliefs and opinions that guide their lives, and they hold onto their opinions in spite of facts that contradict them. A yogini should be able to examine any vritti without attachment. This will not compel her to abandon her beliefs, but it will give her the ability to modify, reject, or retain them.

Insights, Attitudes, and Identification

The causal world is the world of wisdom and insight as well as of infatuation and folly. Insights of a causal nature compel us to re-examine what we once thought was true. An insight might be the realization that someone has been deceiving us, and in that flash of insight a hundred previously unnoticed hints and clues assemble into an obvious picture.

Insights into our personal life are important but essentially self-centered. Artistic and spiritual insights are of a higher causal nature and they are a gift to the world. They are also indicative of spiritual progress. Paradoxically, the loss of concern for a limited self is accompanied by even greater satisfaction. Einstein said that his insight into relativity was one of the most profoundly satisfying events of his life.

The description of causal vrittis as "beliefs and ideas" does not capture all their nuances. Attitudes like pessimism and optimism are causal in nature, and even more profound are our identifications such as the belief that we are a man or a woman or that we are this body. Dr. Motoyama says that when the vrittis that pull a yogini's awareness are of a causal nature, she has progressed very far indeed.

Vrittis and Vasanas

Long suppressed vrittis are called vasanas. Vasanas can lie dormant for years or lifetimes, but when they become active they are more powerful then the presently active vrittis. Dr. Motoyama likens vasanas to inflatable balls being held under water, each ball stacked on top of the other. The further down a ball is held under water, the more violently it will breach the surface.

The top ball of our submerged stack of desires represents our everyday vrittis of work and relationships. Once we dissolve them the next ball of deeper vrittis rises to the surface. Vrittis are not a ceaseless stream, and as we dissolve them we will experience periods of refreshing calm. But when the next submerged vasana rises to the surface it will affect us more strongly than the superficial vrittis of our habitual preoccupations.

An everyday example of the power of vasanas is the midlife crisis. Every significant choice we make compels us to put aside the things not chosen. Our friendships, our schooling, our mating, our chosen profession: all of these choices require us to put aside other options. But at midlife, many of the everyday vrittis that preoccupied us for so long start to lose their power. This is when the suppressed vasanas break onto the surface. Did we choose the right profession? Did we marry the right person? Would we have been more fulfilled if we had pursued these other desires? These emotionally charged vrittis start to haunt us.

Dangers of Chakra Meditation

Vasanas are not rational, but they are powerful. They have seduced smart, successful people into having affairs, leaving their jobs, abandoning their families, and abandoning their spiritual practices. A few years later these people sadly realize that the pain they caused themselves and others was unnecessary and that there were better ways to make these transitions. But vasanas break to the surface with an urgency similar to the impulses of adolescence. It is hard not to be swept away by something that promises to fulfill forgotten longings.

Chakra meditation accelerates the maturation process and takes us through several layers of "midlife crisis." This is the danger of chakra meditation: vasanas make us believe that they represent our real selves, our true desires, and that trying to fulfill them will make us happy at last. But if we examine these vasanas calmly, we will eventually gain the causal insight that these desires are not more uniquely satisfying than our previous desires. This causal insight will slowly absorb the astral energy of the emotionally charged vasanas, and they will dissolve. This absorbed energy now becomes a deeply satisfying and enduring wisdom.

We must be willing to objectively examine all of our beliefs and feelings, and not be attached to them. Every noble and uplifting thought and feeling will easily withstand objective examination. Objective examination of the love I have for my wife does not diminish or dissolve that love, but it will purify it of lingering selfishness. Reflecting on the things we love is called Bhakti Yoga; reflecting on the truths of spiritual teachings is called Jnana Yoga (pronounced gyana yoga).

Summary of Yoga

With so much discussion of nonattachment and dissolving our vasanas, it might seem that yoga is leading us to a dry and desolate place. But this is losing sight of the forest for the trees. Each time we resolve habitual thoughts and emotions, each time we dissolve our attachments, the harvest is greater strength, greater contentment, greater fulfillment, greater wisdom. Nor is yoga a path intended merely to make us content with less.

Now might be a good time to revisit the purpose of yoga as outlined at the beginning of our text.

From ancient times yogis have postulated that there are three levels of human embodiment: a causal body of thought and belief, an astral body of emotion and desire, and a physical body of material substance. Our three bodies are knit together and influence one another through special centers in the spine and brain called chakras. Spiritual adepts assert that our consciousness is not limited to these embodiments and that it can expand beyond them and experience a union with all things in the universe, a union that is fulfilling beyond anything our presently limited existence can offer us. The systematic methods that disentangle our consciousness from our bodies are collectively referred to as the science of yoga. Chakra meditation makes us aware of our emotional attachments and mental misconceptions. If we can patiently dissolve these knots, then our energy and consciousness can slip free of all three bodies and expand into realms of unimagined wisdom and bliss.

CHAPTER 8 Bandha Practices to Awaken Shakti

Shakti and Chi

Chi is constantly circulating through our meridians but the vast potential of Shakti lies dormant in the first chakra at the base of our spine. The relationship between chi and Shakti can be likened to the liquid and solid wax of a burning candle. All the chi presently circulating through the body is like the liquid wax rising up the wick and being burned. The solid wax of the candle is the sleeping Shakti energy being held in reserve.

In traditional language Shakti is said to be sleeping. But sometimes Shakti awakens and infuses us with the energy needed for new or powerful events. A sexual orgasm, the growth of a fetus, and the incredible transformations of puberty are all manifestations of something more than chi, they are manifestations of a partial awakening of Shakti.

The sacred power of Shakti is vital to the tantric yogi. Practicing asana and breathing exercises can harmonize the flow of chi in the meridians, but to open the chakras requires something more than chi—it requires energy of greater strength and subtlety. Shakti must awaken and add her energy to our efforts. Shakti is awakened by intensely focusing our chi into a chakra, bandha practices help to achieve this.

Outline of Bandha Practice

There are several specific muscular contractions that stimulate chi flow around a chakra. These contractions are called Bandhas. Bandha means to restrict or bind.

Bandha practices combine gentle muscular contractions with deep breathing and breath retention. They are usually practiced before meditation, but if a yogini finds her attention wandering during meditation, she might perform bandha practice to refresh and refocus her attention.

Bandha practices gather extra chi into the body and focus it into the area around a chakra and also help to awaken Shakti.

Chakra meditation is subtly fatiguing because breathing is reduced to a low level for a long time. Bandha practices relieve this by bringing extra chi into sushumna, and this allows the yogini to stay comfortably focused for longer periods.

Moving chi continuously in the same pattern will slowly magnetize sushumna. If bandha practices are sustained for a long time, the magnetized sushumna will continue to induce a strong flow of chi even after the bandha practice has ended.

Bandha practices begin by exhaling gently while contracting the muscles that focus chi into the area around a chakra. The inhalation is initiated by releasing the bandha.

Bandha practices are yang, but it is important not to strain. The muscular contractions should be gentle.

Bandha practices are like playing a musical instrument—it is about rhythm and control, not speed and power.

Common rhythms for the number of seconds per exhalation-inhalation-retention are: 4—4—8, 4—4—12, 4—4—16, 8—8—8, or 8—8—16. These numbers are for comparison only. It is not necessary to actually count when breathing.

These suggested rhythms are only approximate, not strict. The essential thing is to find a comfortable rhythm of exhalation—inhalation —retention that is easy to maintain for several minutes.

Do not close the throat (technically the glottis) during retention. Keeping the throat open requires that the yogi maintain an effort as if still inhaling during the retention phase. This creates a continuous flow of energy into the chakra even though no air is being drawn into the lungs.

Muladhara Bandha

In yogic texts this bandha is called mulabandha. The flower of muladhara is the floor of the pelvis, the area that surrounds and supports the anus and genitals. While exhaling, contract the floor of the pelvis and pause for a moment while focused on muladhara. Now release the bandha and guide the inhalation into that area. Hold your breath with your throat open for as long as comfortable. Slowly exhale while contracting the floor of the pelvis. Pause for a moment while focused on muladhara, and then start the next round. Continue in this way for 7, or 14, or 21 repetitions.

During exhalation, contract muladhara bandha and imagine the energies of Shiva and Shakti uniting inside muladhara chakra. During inhalation, imagine Shiva energy descending down sushumna from the top of the head and uniting with Shakti energy inside muladhara at the base of the spine. During retention, imagine the energies of Shiva and Shakti are uniting.

The floor of the pelvis consists of several muscles. Exactly which muscles best stimulate muladhara chakra varies from person to person. A man might contract the muscles of the anus, the perineum, or both. A woman might contract the anus, vaginal muscles, or both. Practice whatever contractions most effectively create tension in the pelvic floor and stimulate awareness of muladhara.

The dominant vasana of muladhara is the desire to exist in this physical world. It is the power that underlies all the other vasanas, which is why this chakra must be awakened. It manifests as identifying with outward things such as our body, possessions, and reputation. To help dissolve and transform these vasanas a yogini should habitually reflect upon her inevitable death. As muladhara opens, the awakened Shakti will give her the power to examine the deeply buried vasanas in all her other chakras.

Svadhisthana Bandha

In yogic texts this bandha is called vajroli. The flower of svadhisthana is the lower abdomen, the area between the navel and pubic bone. While exhaling, contract the lower abdomen and pause for a moment while focused on svadhisthana. Now release the bandha and guide the inhalation into that area. Contract muladhara bandha and hold your breath with your throat open for as long as comfortable. Release muladhara bandha and slowly exhale while contracting the lower abdomen. Pause for a moment while focused on svadhisthana and then start the next round. Continue in this way for 7, or 14, or 21 repetitions.

During exhalation imagine the energies of Shiva and Shakti uniting inside svadhisthana chakra. During inhalation imagine Shiva energy descending sushumna and entering svadhisthana. During retention contract muladhara bandha and imagine Shakti rising up sushumna and uniting with the Shiva energy being held in svadhisthana.

The vasanas of svadhisthana are related to unconscious impulses of lust, anger, and fear. These are typically expressed as overreactions to everyday irritations or as secret or irrational behavior. To help dissolve and transform these vasanas, a yogi should review his daily behaviors and determine if they are in line with his life's goals. Svadhisthana is purified by keeping good company and being honest with oneself. As svadhisthana opens, the yogi stops identifying with his body. This helps him overcome his fears and increases his physical strength.

In the taoist and Zen meditation traditions of China, Korea, and Japan, focus on the hara is of supreme importance. The hara, also called the dan tian, is the area that includes both muladhara and svadhisthana chakras. Dr. Motoyama strongly recommends spending a majority of one's meditation time focused on svadhisthana. Shakti sleeps in muladhara, but when she becomes active she moves into svadhisthana. If svadhisthana is not open, our chi cannot be transmuted into astral or causal energy.

Manipura Bandha

In yogic texts this bandha is called uddiyana. The flower of manipura is the upper abdomen, the area between the navel and the sternum. While exhaling, slowly contract the upper abdomen and pause for a moment while focused on manipura. Now release the bandha and guide the inhalation into that area. Contract muladhara bandha and hold your breath with your throat open for as long as comfortable. Release muladhara bandha and slowly exhale while contracting the upper abdomen. Pause for a moment while focused on manipura, and then start the next round. Continue in this way for 7, or 14, or 21 repetitions.

During exhalation, imagine the energies of Shiva and Shakti uniting inside manipura chakra. During inhalation, imagine Shiva energy descending sushumna and entering manipura. During retention, contract muladhara bandha and imagine Shakti rising up sushumna and uniting with the Shiva energy being held in manipura.

The vasanas of manipura are related to greed and worry. To help dissolve and transform them, a yogini should put aside her judgments and listen to others with compassion. As she transcends her own likes and dislikes, manipura chakra will open and she will be able to clairvoyantly feel other peoples' emotions and intentions. Inwardly she will develop patience and endurance and the ability to hold the body still for a long time.

Anahata Bandha

In yogic texts this bandha is called ujjayi. The flower of anahata is the chest cavity. While exhaling, slightly close the glottis so that the exhaling air creates a soft hissing sound deep in the throat. Now inhale with the glottis still partially closed so that a similar hissing sound is made deep in the throat. Contract muladhara bandha, and hold your breath with your throat open for as long as comfortable. Slowly exhale with ujjayi. Pause for a moment while focused on anahata, and then start the next round. Continue in this way for 7, 14, or 21 repetitions.

During exhalation, imagine the energies of Shiva and Shakti uniting inside anahata chakra. During inhalation, imagine Shiva energy being drawn down sushumna to anahata. During retention, contract muladhara bandha and imagine the energies of Shakti ascending sushumna and uniting with the Shiva energy you are holding in anahata.

Breathing with a partially closed glottis creates a soft hissing sound. It need not be loud or even audible, but in the beginning it is easiest to learn by making an audible hiss deep in the throat.

Remember to take a full inhalation and allow the chest and ribs to expand.

The vasanas of anahata are related to aggression and responsibility. To help dissolve and transform them, the yogi should constantly practice gratitude and contentment. Manipura is the chakra that receives other people's chi, while anahata is the chakra that controls and projects our own chi. As anahata chakra opens, a yogi will develop a healing touch, usually manifest through the hands but also through the voice. He will also be able to effectively move his own chi into his spine and quiet his heart and his breathing. In anahata chakra a yogi finds a restful retreat, a place that the ceaseless sensory noise of the outer world cannot reach.

Vishuddha Bandha

In yogic texts this bandha is called jalandhara. The flower of vishuddha is the throat. Exhale with the same ujjayi breath used for anahata bandha. Now inhale a complete breath while using ujjayi. Close your glottis, contract muladhara bandha, and hold your breath for as long as comfortable. Release muladhara bandha and slowly exhale with ujjayi. Pause for a moment while focused on vishuddha, and then start the next round. Continue in this way for 7, 14, or 21 repetitions.

During exhalation, imagine the energies of Shiva and Shakti uniting inside vishuddha chakra. During inhalation, imagine Shiva energy being drawn down sushumna to vishuddha. During retention, close your glottis, contract muladhara bandha, and imagine the energies of Shakti ascending sushumna and uniting with the Shiva energy you are holding in vishuddha.

Remember to take a full inhalation and allow the chest and ribs to expand.

During retention, relax the abdomen and rib cage so that a gentle pressure is raised against the closed glottis. This is the only bandha where the throat (glottis) is closed during breath retention.

The vasanas of vishuddha are related to pride and grief. To help dissolve and transform them, a yogini should make it a habit to see the beauty in all things and yet recognize that all things are passing. As vishuddha opens, a yogini develops the ability to hold her attention on any subject for long periods of time, and her memory improves. She will also be able to quickly discern between the essential and the nonessential aspects of a person's problems or worries.

Ajna Bandha

Ajna bandha differs from the bandhas of the lower five chakras because it circulates the energies of Shiva and Shakti between muladhara and ajna. These two chakras have a special relationship and the stimulation of one stimulates the other. If muladhara is Shakti's home in the body, then ajna is Shiva's home in the body. Continuously circulating energy between these opposite poles magnetizes all of sushumna and hastens the balanced opening of all chakras.

The root of ajna is the center of the brain and the flower is the front of the brain. The bandha for ajna is the same contraction of the upper abdomen that is used in manipura bandha, but it is used during inhalation rather than exhalation. This creates a slight lifting movement of the rib cage that is not present in manipura bandha. The contraction of the upper abdomen is not a large movement; it is intended to provide resistance to the natural expansion of the upper abdomen.

The bandhas of the first five chakras focus on Shiva descending during inhalation. Ajna bandha focuses on Shakti rising during inhalation. Of course the final goal is to unite both energies at every chakra.

Begin with an exhale while focused on muladhara chakra. Now inhale while slowly contracting the upper abdomen, and imagine drawing Shakti up to ajna chakra. Hold your breath with your throat open for as long as comfortable and imagine Shiva energy descending and uniting with the Shakti being held in ajna. Then exhale slowly as you relax the upper abdomen and imagine the united energies of Shiva and Shakti descending sushumna down to muladhara. Pause for a moment while focused on muladhara, and then start the next round. Continue in this way for 7, 14, or 21 repetitions.

Ajna chakra is the center of wisdom that properly interprets our vasanas and enables us to see through illusions, attachments, and misconceptions. It is the chakra through which the yogini makes contact with higher spiritual powers, and if it is not open then she is in danger of being swept away by the vasanas that are activated in the five lower chakras.

To help awaken ajna chakra a yogi should make it a habit to pause several times a day and listen to the nada of ajna.

Variations of Ajna Bandha

Variations of ajna bandha are some of the most important practices of tantric and taoist meditation. A text in the taoist tradition entitled "The Secret of the Golden Flower" proclaims that no other technique is necessary for a yogi. Paramahansa Yogananda (1893-1952), a twentieth-century Indian yogi, was of the same opinion, and in his writings emphasized variations of ajna bandha that he called Kriya Yoga.

Taoist versions of ajna bandha are referred to as "Circulation of Light" or "Reverse Breathing." In taoist practices the path of energy circulation is not typically described as up and down sushumna, it is described as an orbit "up the back of the body" and "down the front of the body." In my experience, energy moves both within sushumna and along the front and back of the body. I believe the energy felt nearer the body surface is chi, and the energy felt within sushumna is Shiva-Shakti energy. I also believe both types of energy flow influence each other. Moving energy up the back of the body and down the front of the body influences the energy within sushumna, just like an electric current moving around an iron bar will magnetize it.

Circulation of Light

This version of ajna bandha brings energy up the back of the body and down the front. This practice uses both muladhara bandha and manipura bandha during the inhalation phase, muladhara bandha starts the inhalation and manipura bandha completes it. Start with an exhalation while bringing the energy of ajna chakra down the front of the body to svadhisthana. Pause for a moment and contract muladhara bandha. Then release muladhara bandha to start the inhalation. Continue inhaling while gently contracting manipura bandha, this helps draw the energy up to ajna chakra. Hold your breath with your throat open for as long as comfortable while focused on ajna chakra. Exhale to start the next cycle. During inhalation, the energy first descends from svadhisthana to muladhara and is then drawn up the back of the body to ajna chakra.

Reverse Breathing

This version of ajna bandha brings energy up the front of the body and down the back. Start with an exhalation while bringing the energy of ajna chakra down the back of the body to muladhara chakra. Pause for a moment, then inhale with manipura bandha and draw the energy up the front of the body to ajna chakra. Hold your breath with your throat open for as long as comfortable and then exhale while bringing the energy down the back of the body to muladhara chakra.

Sahasrara Bandha

Sahasrara bandha is unique among the bandhas as it attempts to lift Shakti up through sushumna and out of the body. Sahasrara bandha purifies sushumna and is particularly helpful after meditation. The effort of concentration can sometimes stagnate chi in the head and create uncomfortable stuffiness or pressure. Sahasrara bandha opens Brahman's Gate at the top of the head and allows this excess chi a natural path of escape.

Brahman's Gate is the opening at the top of the head, but it is neither the root nor the flower of sahasrara chakra. The root of sahasrara is the top of the brain and the flower is imagined as a point in space above the head. The opening in the top of the head is a gate through which the energy passes, but it does not reside there.

The bandha for sahasrara is the same contraction of the upper abdomen that is used in manipura bandha, but the bandha is applied during inhalation rather than exhalation. This creates a slight lifting movement of the rib cage that is not present in manipura bandha. The contraction of the upper abdomen is not a large movement; it is intended to provide resistance to the natural expansion of the upper abdomen.

The bandhas of the first five chakras focus on Shiva descending during inhalation. Sahasrara bandha focuses on Shakti rising during inhalation.

Begin with an exhale while focused on muladhara chakra. Now inhale while slowly contracting the upper abdomen, and imagine drawing Shakti up sushumna and out through the top of your head. Hold your breath with your throat open for as long as comfortable and imagine the energy of Shiva surrounding and uniting with the Shakti you are holding in the space above you. Then exhale slowly as you relax your upper abdomen. Imagine the united energies of Shiva and Shakti descending through the top of your head and down sushumna to muladhara. Pause for a moment while focused on muladhara, and then start the next round. Continue in this way for 7, 14, or 21 repetitions.

Some yogis imagine raising their Shakti a foot or two above their head. Others imagine it rising to great distances. Experiment to see which imaginative effort best stirs the movement of your energy and awareness.

Our beliefs determine how we judge the events of our life. How we judge the events of our life determines how we react to them, and these reactions determine our pleasurable and painful experiences in this life as well as the vasanas for this and future lives. Our strongest limiting belief is that our body is the basis of our existence, and it colors all other judgments. There is really no cure for this until we consciously experience a state of existence beyond the body. Sahasrara is the gate through which a yogini must consciously pass to experience existence beyond the body.

To help awaken sahasrara chakra a yogini should imagine herself rising out of Brahman's Gate and try to feel her body is inside her consciousness rather than feel her consciousness is inside her body.

CHAPTER **9** Pranayama
Practices

Yang Pranayama as an Alternative to Bandha Practice

Some yogins do not like the muscular effort of bandha practices, even though these efforts are gentle. Other yogins find the visualizations of Shiva and Shakti energy movement distracting, especially as a beginner. These yogins might prefer to use a more general yang pranayama to focus the mind and gather chi into the chakras.

Indian yogis tell us that the vibration of inhalation is very much like the vibration of the syllable *so*, and that the vibration of exhalation is very much like the syllable *ham*. *So* rhymes with *toe* and *ham* rhymes with *thumb*. Taken together these syllables are the SoHam mantra. Yang pranayama uses this mantra to lengthen and deepen the breath and this gathers more chi into a chakra. Yang pranayama is practiced as follows.

Focus on a chakra and inhale while mentally chanting the mantra So. Draw out the syllable as a long soooooooooo for the duration of the inhalation, which should last from four to eight seconds. Hold your breath with your throat open for as long as comfortable. Then exhale while mentally chanting the mantra Ham. Draw out the syllable as a long hammmmmmm for the duration of the exhalation, which should last four to eight seconds. Repeat 7, 14, or 21 times.

There is a yin and a yang to everything and yang pranayama is no exception. Yang pranayama can also be done while chanting the syllable *ham* on the inhalation and the syllable *sa* on the exhalation. *Ham* rhymes with *thumb* and *sa* rhymes with *saw*. This mantra is called HamSa and it is the yang version of SoHam. It is used as follows.

Focus on a chakra and inhale while mentally chanting Ham. Draw out the syllable for the duration of the inhalation, which should last four to eight seconds. Hold your breath with your throat open for as long as comfortable. Then exhale while mentally chanting Sa. Draw out the syllable for the duration of the exhalation, which should last four to eight seconds. Repeat 7, 14, or 21 times.

Using the SoHam mantra helps the descent of chi and Shiva energy down the spine. Using the HamSa mantra helps draw chi and Shakti up the spine. A yogin must experiment to determine which mantra works best on each chakra. I habitually use SoHam for the three lower chakras and HamSa for the four higher chakras.

Breath in Three Dimensions

The first step in chakra purification is to conserve the chi of the physical body and this is achieved by sitting still and reducing the breath. But all three bodies interpenetrate each other and breathing is more than physical. Yoga teaches that our thoughts, emotions and breath are intimately connected. If our breathing is restless or uneven, it reflects an emotional or distracted mind, and if the breathing is subtle and slow, it reflects a calm and concentrated mind. It is also true that if we quiet our physical breath we will calm and focus our astral and causal energies.

Three Phases of Normal Breathing

There are three phases to normal breathing: inhalation, exhalation, and neutral. You can easily observe these phases by calmly watching your breathing for a few minutes. Watch with a yin attitude, the attitude of a naturalist. Do not try to alter your breathing, just calmly observe the three phases.

The first phase is an automatic inhalation, a gentle expansion of the abdomen or ribs that is controlled by the autonomic nervous system. Inhalation is almost immediately followed by a passive exhalation. This exhalation is considered passive because no muscular effort is required to exhale—the natural elasticity of the ribs and abdomen gently force the air out of the lungs as they contract back to their neutral position.

During the neutral phase there is no urge to inhale or exhale. This phase lasts for several seconds or more depending on how calm you are. After this neutral pause, the next inhalation will begin and the cycle continues. All of this happens without our conscious interference.

Yin Pranayama

The goal of yin pranayama is to effortlessly extend the neutral phase of the breath cycle. This is very different from yang pranayama, the goal of which is to extend breath retention after inhalation. Yin pranayama uses the same SoHam or HamSa mantras that are used in yang pranayama, but they are used in a very different way. Yin pranayama is practiced as follows.

Focus on a chakra and wait for the natural inhalation to arise. Mentally chant So when the inhalation begins, and mentally chant Ham when the exhalation begins. These mantras are mentally chanted just once and their pronunciation is not extended as they are in yang pranayama. Inhalation and exhalation gradually become very brief and very shallow, and the neutral phase grows longer and longer. It is important not to hold the breath or resist inhaling, just stay focused on the chakra and sink into the quiet state of not breathing.

There is a yin and a yang to everything and yin pranayama is no exception. Yin pranayama can also be done with the HamSa mantra rather than the SoHam mantra. Breathing with HamSa follows the same pattern as SoHam but the yogi mentally chants Ham on the inhalation and Sa on the exhalation.

The use of SoHam and HamSa effect the sensation of a chakra much like the diastole and systole phases of the heart beat. The effect of each mantra is felt most powerfully during inhalation. Mentally chanting So on the inhalation creates an expanding feeling around a chakra. Mentally chanting Ham on the inhalation creates a contracting feeling around a chakra. Experiment with both to become familiar with their effects. This is the only way to intelligently decide which mantra is appropriate on any given day.

10 Meditation

Listening to Nada

The common thread to all phases of yoga practice is controlling chi with increasingly subtle techniques. Starting with asana exercises and physical stillness, yoga then progresses to the gentle muscular contractions of bandhas, and then to the more subtle yang pranayama, and then to the even more subtle yin pranayama. The next phase of practice is beyond the breath, it is listening to internal sounds called Nada.

The act of listening quiets the breath and the mind. Try this exercise: Pause for a moment and focus on a sound that is quiet, almost inaudible, perhaps a quiet hum in your room or a muffled sound from outside. Whatever it is, observe that as you listen you unconsciously suspend your breathing. The more subtle the sound the quieter the breath becomes. Yogis have taken this principle to its subtlest level and prescribe that students focus on sounds that can only be heard within themselves, sounds created by the vibrating chakras. These sounds are called Nada. To learn to hear nada, try the following exercise.

Rest your middle three fingers on your temples rest the little fingers lightly on the outer corners of your closed eyes. This will inhibit eye movement and assist a calm focus. Now use your thumbs to press the tragus into your ears (the tragus is the small flap of cartilage nearly covering the ear canal). Now listen to sounds arising from inside your ears. The right ear is said to be more sensitive, but with practice it will make no difference which ear you focus with, just listen for sounds.

When you focus on nada as a meditation it is not necessary to use your hands or press the tragus into your ears. With practice you can hear the nada whenever you are in a quiet place and focus your awareness.

Nadas of the Chakras

Each of the chakras has a unique nada sound that is tabulated below. In my experience each chakra has a small range of nada sounds, but there is a marked difference between the nada of one chakra and another. Bear in mind that these traditional descriptions can only crudely approximate the actual sounds. What a yogini hears in meditation is difficult to describe, but these approximations do help her decipher what she is hearing.

CHAKRA	NADA SOUND
Sahasrara	Om Sound
Ajna	Om Sound
Vishuddha	Ocean
Anahata	Deep Bell
Manipura	Harp Strings
Svadhisthana	Flute
Muladhara	Buzzing Bees

Nada Meditation

Yin pranayama seamlessly blends into Nada Meditation. Start your meditation with yin pranyama and as you get quiet listen for nada. These techniques are not mutually exclusive and it is perfectly fine to continue yin pranayama while listening to nada. As time passes, let go of breath-awareness and focus only on nada. If your attention wavers, resume yin pranayama until you are calm, and then slip into nada again.

After listening to nada for a while you will become aware of two or more competing sounds. Continue to calmly focus on whichever is the most obvious nada until it fades, and then focus on the next nada that becomes apparent.

Different chakras are more dominant than others, so do not assume that the nada you are hearing is emanating from the chakra on which you are focused. It is possible the nada is coming from another chakra that is more active at this time. Only a highly advanced meditator can selectively experience the nada of the chakra of her choosing.

Nyasa Ritual

It is good to begin and end meditation with nyasa. Nyasa means "to place within." There are several variations of nyasa practice, some simple, some elaborate. They effectively prepare us for chakra meditation.

Open your meditation by imagining the vastness of the consciousness of Shiva, a consciousness that extends to all parts of the universe in all dimensions of existence. Imagine this consciousness condensing and descending down into your body, stopping briefly at each chakra until united with Shakti at the base of the spine. Enjoy this union of consciousness and energy for a while, and then begin your meditation.

End your practice by drawing your energy and awareness into muladhara, then imagine yourself rising with Shakti up through sushumna one chakra at a time, and then out through the top of your head. Continue rising and expanding until you dissolve into Shiva.

Bija mantras

Nyasa practice can be assisted by bija mantras. Bija means "seed" and bija mantras are simple sound vibrations that stimulate specific chakras. When focusing on a chakra, mentally chant its bija mantra and feel its response. Repeat the mantra as many times as you wish, and then move on to the next chakra.

The bija mantras for each chakra are as follows:

Sahasrara	Om	Rhymes with home
Ajna	Om	Rhymes with home
Vishuddha	Ham	Rhymes with thumb
Anahata	Yam	Rhymes with thumb
Manipura	Ram	Rhymes with thumb
Svadhisthana	Vam	Rhymes with thumb
Muladhara	Lam	Rhymes with thumb

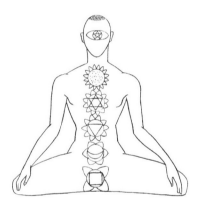

Bija Meditation

I frequently use a variation of nyasa practice as my primary meditation. Using bija mantras, I circulate my awareness and energy up and down sushumna one chakra at a time. Each cycle takes approximately two minutes to complete and I practice for 7, 14, or 21 cycles.

Throughout this practice I remain focused on nada and when I finish the cycles of circulation I remain absorbed in nada for as long as possible.

Meditation Routine

The following is an outline for a beginning meditation practice of about fifteen minutes.

1. One minute opening nyasa practice ending at muladhara.
2. Seven rounds of bandha practice or yang pranayama for one chakra.
3. Five minutes yin pranayama on that chakra.
4. Five minutes of nada meditation on that chakra.
5. One minute closing nyasa practice ending above the head.

Suggestions for Meditation

I suggest that beginners focus on only one chakra every day for a week, and keep a diary of your experiences. Then focus on another chakra each day for one week. In seven weeks you will have meditated on each of the seven chakras.

Once you have explored each chakra you might repeat the cycle of focusing on one chakra each week, or you might try focusing on a different chakra each day.

After a few months, try to expand your meditation to include more bandha practice and longer nada meditation.

If your meditation or pranayama practices create tension or discomfort, then something is wrong. Think of doing your practices as if you were a child going to school. It obviously requires some discipline to progress, but if every day at school created discomfort, then progress would eventually stop and the child's soul would whither rather than blossom.

Bibliography

Books on Anatomy

Thomas W. Myers, *Anatomy Trains: Myofascial Meridians for Manual and Movement Therapists, Second Edition,* (Churchill Livingston, Philadelphia, 2008).
Fascia is not given enough emphasis in standard textbooks. This book corrects that deficiency. It is an extensive discussion of the prevalence of fascia and its influence on movement and movement pathology. The illustrations alone can lead a yogi or body worker into numerous "aha!" moments.

Deane Juhan, *Job's Body: A Handbook for Bodywork,* (Station Hill, Barrytown, NY, 2003).
The classic and in most ways unsurpassed description of how fascia integrates all the systems of the body and why touching and massaging the body has such healing effects.

Michael Schuenke et al., *Thieme Atlas of Anatomy: General Anatomy and the Musculoskeletal System*, (Thieme, New York, 2010).
This is part one of a three-volume atlas. It is especially useful for yogis because it combines the muscles and bones of anatomy with charts that illustrate the different movements of each muscle group. The pictures are gorgeous and the many graphs and schematic charts are invaluable and not readily available elsewhere. This atlas was written with the eager student in mind, unlike most reference works.

Andrew Biel, *Trail Guide to the Body: How to Locate Muscles, Bones, and More*, (Books of Discovery, Boulder, CO, 2010).
This is an excellent guide to learning how to feel through the skin and locate the structures that are pictured in anatomy texts. It is literally the hands-on approach to anatomy that a teacher or body worker needs.

Leslie Kaminoff and Amy Matthews, *Yoga Anatomy*, (Human Kinetics, Champaign, IL, 2010).
This hugely popular book on the anatomy of muscles and bones shows how the muscles are worked in a variety of yoga poses. This is much more helpful to a yoga student than the static "corpse position" of standard anatomy texts.

Books on Acupuncture

Joseph M. Helms, *Acupuncture Energetics: A Clinical Approach for Physicians*, (Medical Acupuncture Publishers, Berkeley, 1995).
Chinese medicine and acupuncture are vast subjects that include herbs, diagnosis, needling technique, and so on. What is most relevant to a yogini is where the meridians are and how they influence one another. This is the best resource I have found for cogently and clearly identifying the meridians and their functional groups. In many ways this book is acupuncture's response to the *Thieme Atlas of Anatomy* described above. It takes great skill and insight to create charts and schematics that accurately clarify a confusing body of facts, and this book is full of them. Obviously written by a master teacher.

Claudia Focks, ed., *Atlas of Acupuncture*, (Churchill Livingston, Philadelphia, 2008).
This stunningly complete atlas collates the work of most of the atlases of acupuncture now in print. Its mix of photographs and illustration will make it a standard reference book on points and meridians for years to come.

Edward F. Tarabilda, *Ayurveda Revolutionized: Integrating Ancient and Modern Ayurveda*, (Lotus Press, Twin Lakes, WI, 1997).
Ayurveda is the ancient medical tradition of India, but like any form of medicine it has gone through many developments and changes in the thousands of years of its existence. Tarabilda argues that although many of the basic notions of ayurveda are correct, several key ideas on how to apply them effectively have been lost. He reconstructs several of these key ideas based on his original insights into Vedic astrology. One aspect of these insights is the reintegration of meridian theory into ayurvedic energetics.

James L. Oschman, *Energy Medicine in Therapeutics and Human Performance*, (Buterworth-Heinemann, Philadelphia, 2003).
Not really an acupuncture book, but it is included because it is a 350-page discussion of the ways in which modern research is confirming and expanding on the basic insights of yoga and acupuncture theory. Chapters on cells, fascia, waterflow, liquid crystals, electrical and magnetic signaling, and more are described and illustrated with pictures and drawings. Oschman spells out very clearly the implications of this research and the new view of biology that is just around the corner. If you are interested in what modern science has to say about ancient science, this book is for you.

Books on Yoga Asana

Bernie Clark, *The Complete Guide to Yin Yoga: The Philosophy and Practice of Yin Yoga*, (White Cloud Press, Ashland, OR, 2012).
The strongest recommendation I can give Bernie's book is to say it is a textbook for my own training programs. The first section outlines the philosophy of yin-yang, the second section details each pose, and the third section explains the science behind the practice. Students value its clear, logical outline of yoga and the relevant anatomical discussion.

Swami Muktibodhananda, *Hatha Yoga Pradipika*, (Bihar School of Yoga, Bihar, India, 1998).
This is a modern commentary on an old text of hatha yoga. The ancient text is only 400 verses long, but this elaboration is over 700 pages. A serious student of any subject should know something of its foundational texts, and this one is key. A modern yogi might be shocked to learn how little emphasis is placed on asana practice. Most of the original hatha yoga practices are pranayama and purification practices. The goal was to awaken the chakra by purifying the meridians and becoming absorbed into nada. Nada meditation is emphasized as the key to reaching the highest states of yoga.

Sarah Powers, *Insight Yoga*, (Shambhala, Boston, 2008).
Sarah Powers integrates yin and yang yoga with mindfulness practices, and this three-legged approach makes her book a truly complete yoga system, not just a yin system. Powers includes detailed descriptions of meridian pathways and how they are related to yoga poses. This helps connect the practice of yoga to disciplines such as shiatsu, acupuncture, and bodywork. Integration with other disciplines is key to yoga's broader acceptance into the modern world, and this book is a natural starting point for interested yoginis.

B. K. S. Iyengar, *Light on Yoga: Yoga Dipika*, (Schocken Books, New York, 1995).
Every serious student of yoga needs a reference book of postures, and this one is it. There are others, but none are really better. There are more postures listed here than most students will need, but that is the function of a reference book. The step-by-step descriptions of each pose have never really been surpassed.

Cheri Clampett and Biff Mithoefer, *The Therapeutic Yoga Kit: Sixteen Postures for Self-Healing through Quiet Yin Awareness*, (Healing Arts Press, Rochester, VT, 2009).
If I were injured or recovering from illness, this is the system and these are the teachers I would start with. Clampett and Mithoefer have honestly and humbly tested these techniques for years. Their students range from people who are injured to the aged to cancer ward patients. The combination of book, flashcards, and CD make it possible for even beginning students to safely learn these techniques.

Biff Mithoefer, *The Yin Yoga Kit: The Practice of Quiet Power*, (Healing Arts Press, Rochester, VT, 2006).
Biff Mithoefer has taught and practiced yoga for decades. As everyone knows, a teacher can make or break a student's interest in the early phase of study, and Mithoefer is one of the good ones. He teaches energetic principles of chi and meridians and integrates them with asanas and mindfulness. The use of a book, flashcards, and CD is extremely effective for a self-learner.

Books on Meditation and Spirituality

Paramahansa Yogananda, *Autobiography of a Yogi*, (Self-Realization Fellowship, Los Angeles, 2000).
This is a personal book about the life and goals of a yogi. One man's experience cannot illustrate every aspect of yoga, but yoga is the most personal of experiences. Not only is the science of yoga discussed at length, but the footnotes can lead the reader into many rewarding areas of scientific, historical, and religious study.

Hiroshi Motoyama, *Awakening of the Chakras and Emancipation*, (Human Science Press, Encinitas, CA, 2003).
Based on talks given to advanced meditators, this book details the postures, pranayamas, and concentration exercises Dr. Motoyama recommends for each chakra. It includes descriptions of what to expect at the physical, astral, and causal levels of chakra awakening, as well as the signs of proper progress and the signs of improper practice. This is the most detailed description of chakra meditation of which I am aware.

Paramahansa Yogananda, *God Talks with Arjuna: The Bhagavad Gita*, (Self-Realization Fellowship, Los Angeles, 2001).
The first one hundred pages of this thousand-page commentary on the Bhagavad Gita integrates the teachings of the Gita, Samkhya philosophy, and Patanjali's sutras. It is a colossal intellectual and spiritual achievement. If any of these subjects interest you, consider this two-volume work.

Rudolf Steiner, *How to Know Higher Worlds*, (Wilder Publications, Radford, VA, 2008).
This book outlines the spiritual practices of Dr. Steiner. It includes detailed psychological descriptions of the chakras and their usefulness in spiritual practice. It is always worthwhile to read about chakras from a variety of backgrounds and traditions.

Hiroshi Motoyama, *Karma and Reincarnation: The Key to Spiritual Evolution and Enlightenment*, (Avon Books, 2008).
More simple and direct than many of Dr. Motoyama's works, this book is about the varieties of karma that affect us. Karma is not just personal—there is also family karma, land karma, national karma, and the influence of greater spiritual beings.

Swami Vivekananda, *Raja Yoga*, (Ramakrishna-Vivekananda Center, New York, 1980).
Patanjali is the codifier of yoga meditation. His succinctly written book has guided yogis and attracted scholarly commentary for centuries. This book is a clear introduction to Patanjali's system. It includes several preliminary lectures that set the stage for Patanjali's work, as well as the great swami's version of the sutras. It takes a good teacher to make the material clear and Swami Vivekananda is a teacher for the ages.

Paramahansa Yogananda, *The Science of Religion*, (Self-Realization Fellowship, Los Angeles, 1953).
An expansion of Swami Yogananda's first talk in America, this book is especially helpful in delineating the difference between the four paths to enlightenment, and the unique characteristics of yoga.

Richard Wilhelm, translator. C. G. Jung, commentary, *Secret of the Golden Flower: A Chinese Book of Life*, (Harcourt & Brace, New York, 1962).
This is a translation and commentary on the ancient variation of ajna bandha, herein called "Circulation of the Light." Wilhelm has clarified the meaning of the deliberately flowery language used to describe the practice. A dedicated student will find the technique familiar and the noble sentiments inspiring.

Hiroshi Motoyama, *Theories of the Chakras: Bridge to Higher Consciousness*, (Quest Books, Wheaton, IL, 1982).
This book was written to fulfill three objectives: demonstrate that tantric and taoist yogis were describing the same energy system; detail a series of practices to awaken the chakras; and report on the scientific investigation of chi, meridians, and chakras. This was my first introduction to Dr. Motoyama's valuable contribution to the future of energy medicine and spiritual practice.

Rudolf Steiner, *Theosophy: An Introduction to the Spiritual Processes in Human Life and in the Cosmos*, (Anthroposophic Press, Hudson, NY, 1994).

This book outlines Dr. Steiner's views of the different bodies we inhabit. It is illuminating to read about the multiple body theory from a European mystic's viewpoint. It is always encouraging to have phenomena confirmed by different practitioners from different traditions. This is the essence of the scientific method.

Hiroshi Motoyama, *Varieties of Mystical Experience*, (Human Science Press, Encinitas, CA, 2006).
If *Awakening of the Chakras and Emancipation* describes the techniques of practice, this book describes the goal. It is a description of the various levels of samadhi, the state of spiritual union with higher beings. It goes into great detail about how our consciousness changes as we enter into higher spiritual states of awareness. It makes clear what our attitude and motivation should be if we wish to consciously progress. This is a mind-expanding and inspiring book.

Swami Hariharananda Aranya, *Yoga Philosophy of Patanjali*, (SUNY Press, Albany, NY, 1984).
This is the book for philosophers. If Vivekananda is the popularizer of Patanjali, then Hariharananda is Patanjali's meticulous analyst. Hariharananda was a dedicated practitioner, and his analysis of each sutra is not meant to be pedantic but rather to uncover its explicit psychological and spiritual meaning. The premise of the book is an ancient one, that the sutras were meant to be the practical application of the ancient samkhya philosophy. Studying this text means absorbing the ideas of samkhya as well as yoga, and this is what makes the book so rewarding to the dedicated student.

Edwin F. Bryant, *The Yoga Sutras of Patanjali: A New Edition, Translation, and Commentary*, (North Point Press, New York, 2009).
There are many translations of Patanjali, and this latest one is excellent in many ways, not the least of which is the presentation of how commentators on the sutras have spoken to each other over the centuries. Being exposed to different peoples' reactions to the same material makes us re-examine our own. After reading *Raja Yoga* by Vivekananda, this book is the next step.

Appendix

Yin yoga is a new name, but not a new practice. With few exceptions, yoga practice before the ashtanga vinyasa revolution of 1980s was primarily yin. The quotes listed below are from four yoga books, one for each decade prior to 1985. They were all written by authors considered authorities in the field. Each quote includes a few example poses, the recommended time for holding them, and the yin attitude that was recommended when practicing.

Hatha Yoga by Theos Bernard
Rider and Company, 1950

Seal: 1 minute 10 times
Caterpillar: 1 minute 10 times or for several minutes.
Snail: Up to 10 minutes

Yin attitude defined: "I was satisfied to place my hands on my ankles and let my head come as close to the knees as was comfortable without forcing it." (p. 26)

Hatha Yoga by Shyam Sundar Goswami
L.N. Fowler and Company, 1959

Seal: 6 minutes.
Caterpillar: 6 minutes.
Snail: 15 minutes

Yin attitude defined: "In the static form of exercise the whole body. . . should remain absolutely motionless. . . for the period of time during which the posture can be maintained with ease, i.e. without the feeling of discomfort." (pp. 80-81)

Yoga Self-Taught by André Van Lysebeth
Harper and Row, 1971

Seal: several minutes
Caterpillar: 3 to 15 minutes.
Snail: 5 to 30 minutes.

Yin attitude defined: "The expert keeps a perpetual check on muscular relaxation . . . everything relaxes: the face, arms, hands, feet, calves, thighs, and especially the muscles that are being stretched." (p. 73)

The Sivananda Companion to Yoga by Lucy Lidell
Simon and Schuster, 1983

Back Bends: 2 minutes
Forward Bends: 5 minutes
Inversions: 5 to 10 minutes

Yin attitude defined: "Above all, never risk injury by forcing your body into a position or straining to go further than you are presently able. It is only when your muscles are relaxed that they will stretch and allow you to advance in a posture." (p. 29)

About the Author

Paul and Suzee Grilley have been teaching yoga since 1980. They practice yoga postures in the style of Paulie Zink and pattern their philosophy on the writings and research of Dr. Hiroshi Motoyama. This philosophy integrates the meridian theories of China with the chakra theories of India. Paul and Suzee have developed the anatomically based Yin Yoga Teacher Training program which they present all over the world.

To learn more about their work; books, DVDs, and other resources, please visit www.paulgrilley.com.

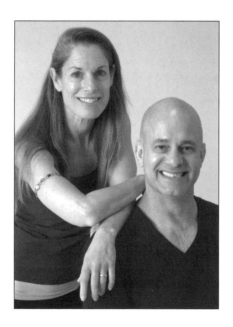

Yoga and Eastern Wisdom
from White Cloud Press

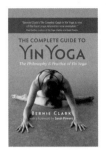

THE COMPLETE GUIDE TO YIN YOGA
The Philosophy & Practice of Yin Yoga
BERNIE CLARK, FOREWORD BY SARAH POWERS
$18.95 / Yoga / ISBN: 978-1-935952-50-3

"Bernie Clark's Complete Guide to Yin Yoga is one of the best yoga resources now available." Paul Grilley

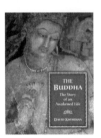

THE BUDDHA The Story of an Awakened Life
BY DAVID KHERDIAN
$14.95 / Buddhism / ISBN: 978-1-883991-63-0

Here is a simple, elegant introduction to the Buddha's path, in which you may "work out your salvation with diligence."

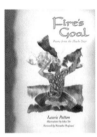

FIRE'S GOAL Poems from the Hindu Year
BY LAURIE PATTON, PH.D, ILLUSTRATIONS BY LIKA TOV
$14.95 / Hinduism / Poetry / ISBN: 978-1-883991-49-4

These poems reflect a year of journeys to sacred river sources in India. Patton's poems were written after a decade of writing and reading interpretations of India's most sacred Sanskrit compositions—the Vedas.

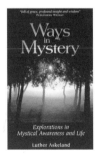

WAYS IN MYSTERY
Explorations in Mystical Awareness and Life
BY LUTHER ASKELAND
$17 / Mysticism / 978-1883991-16-6

"Ranging across the teachings of the masters of the mystical tradition—Christian mystics St. John of the Cross and Meister Eckhart; Buddhist sage Nagajuna; Zen Master Dogen and Tanzen; Indian saint Shankara—Askeland works to recover the mystical path known as the way of unknowing. Askeland here seeks to recapture an authentic spirituality, and understanding of God that exceeds all speech and thought. His essays are full of grace, profound insight and wisdom." Publishers Weekly

For more information on these and other spiritual books, visit our website: whitecloudpress.com